FOOD
FOR
FITNESS

Published by
World Publications

Copyright ⓔ 1975 by BIKE WORLD MAGAZINE

First Printing - January 1975
Second Printing - April 1976
Third Printing - December 1976
Fourth Printing - June 1977
Fifth Printing - November 1977

Library of Congress Catalog Card Number: 74-16792

ISBN: 0-89037-053-2

WORLD PUBLICATIONS, P.O. Box 366, Mt. View, CA 94040

Cover trophy compliments of F & S Bowling and Trophy Supply, Mt. View, California

CONTENTS

FOREWORD

"My body works OK, it turns in good times, it doesn't get bellyaches—so what's wrong with what I eat?" If you think this way, or tend to, this booklet will help you understand the bad effects of wrong eating on your athletic performance and just feeling good, and the positive ground you can gain by good diet—in performance and feeling *great*. In fact, we're quite confident you'll get your money's worth in results out of *Food for Fitness*.

Very little has been published on the best fuels for the athletic "machine," and we've just about drained all our nutritional resources as a publishing company with seven (or is it eight now?) sports magazines edited by and for the participant. A lot *has* been done in the field of performance nutrition, only it's never before been made available to the athlete with no time to dig into research papers and the literature of general nutrition.

Since written records began there have been two schools of health—one of curing and one of hygiene. The medical profession and its enormous twin, the drug industry, are the modern versions of the school of curing. We as athletes are interested in much more than curing or preventing disease: our goal is to get to even higher levels of functional efficiency and disease-free positive vitality. The nutritional stance of medical science has been: "Wait until the lab boys come up with something—then we'll believe it's worthwhile." As Dr. Ralph Bircher points out, the laboratory conclusions "contradict so fantastically that the reader finds himself holding his head in despair."

We found ourselves increasingly convinced by the thinking of Dr. Otto Brucker's "new nutritionists." "You can't improve on Mother Nature's finished product," these avant garde researchers say. At the same time, we've presented the facts as we found them, not compromising to pamper private or social tastes, customs or conveniences.

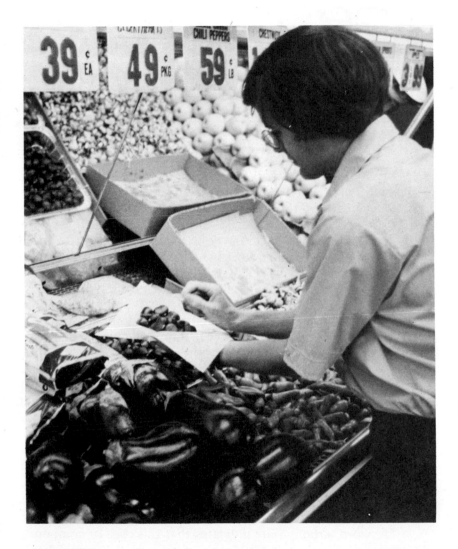

1

The Athlete's Diet

by Dr. Creig Hoyt

After the brilliant work at the turn of the century on vitamin deficiencies and related diseases the science of nutrition became increasingly divorced from modern medical concerns. However, events of the last few years suggesting that heart disease is related to diet, that the common cold may be prevented by mega-doses of vitamin C, and that refined sugars and starches may be responsible for increasing rates of cancer of the bowel are only a sampling of the topics of current debate in clinical medicine circles.

Elsewhere in this book you will find reports championing various diets or supplements. I agree with some of these and disagree with others. However, in order to provide you with a better framework from which to evaluate these other reports, I shall attempt to present a non-partisan survey of what is accepted by most nutritional experts today as established data concerning nutrition and exercise. In so doing, I shall discuss the role of proteins, fats and carbohydrates (their requirements, toxic effects and specific limitations or advantages in sports). I shall then turn to a similar brief review of vitamins and trace minerals. I shall not attempt to synthesize the "ideal" athletic diet, but rather provide you with the information necessary to construct your own diet.

CARBOHYDRATES

The word carbohydrate indicates that this class of compounds is composed of carbon and hydrogen/oxygen in the same 2:1 ratio as in water. They may be either simple sugars (glucose, fructose or galactose) or more complex molecules of many units of these simple sugars—starches. Nevertheless, their primary role whether as sugars or starches is to supply a quick, cheap source of energy.

Muscles prefer carbohydrates during strenuous exercise due to their efficient metabolism. Although the liver does store carbohydrates in the form of glycogen, this can be exhausted easily in exercise like bike races of 50 miles or more. It is for this reason that most athletes eat carbohydrates during such strenuous rides and/or "carbohydrate load" for several days before the activity. Other advantages to carbohydrates are their quick transit time through the gut (compared to fats and proteins), making them easier to digest while exercising, and the significant water supply that they provide when broken down through digestion. Obviously, their benefit in hot weather is unchallenged due to their water content. Thus, carbohydrates are the preferred mainstay both during and just before a race, game or training session.

However, it should be noted that for the non-exercising individual the only real advantage of carbohydrates is their relatively low cost per calories supplied. They are not essential for the sedentary diet. They provide no essential intermediary compounds, nor bind any vitamins. And while it is true that the brain requires carbohydrates for normal metabolism, the body can if necessary generate enough carbohydrate from fat stores (a process known as gluconeogenesis).

Thus, we see the paradoxical situation with carbohydrates—they are not absolutely necessary for the normal diet, but to the active athlete they become his major source of energy. There have been postulations from some medical centers that the increased consumption of refined sugars and starches is related to atherosclerosis (hardening of the arteries) and bowel cancer. Neither of these two theories have been proven, but they warrant concern and consideration. There are no definite requirements for carbohydrates, nor is there a specific level of carbohydrates most conducive to good health, but the above factors should be weighed when you decide on how much and what type of carbohydrates to include in your diet.

FATS

Fats, like carbohydrates, contain carbon, hydrogen and oxygen. However, the hydrogen content varies according to how "saturated" the fat is: the hydrogen to oxygen ratio is not 2:1 as it is in carbohydrates. Because of fats' low oxygen content they have a very high calorie value per weight. On a weight basis, fats provide nearly 2½ times as many calories as carbohydrates. Fats are found in both plants and animals. Indeed, this is the big worry among many cardiologists—our high fat intake is related to our current pandemic of vascular disorders. The average American diet obtains 40-45% of calories from fats; most researchers believe that 25% would be much more helpful. Part of the problem is that we have developed tastes that cater to hidden fat contents; for example, if you trim all the visible fat from a steak it will still be 10–12% fat. We often forget about the fats we use in cooking, in sauces, in dressings. Fats are not inherently harmful. In fact, they have a more essential role in nutrition than do carbohydrates.

The body requires a minimum amount of essential fatty acids to maintain health and growth. If this is not provided, the body will lose tissue viability—especially in the kidneys and skin. Secondly, fats are the carriers of fat-soluble vitamins (A, D, E, K). One could, of course, get these in supplement forms, but it is more practical and efficient to obtain them in the diet. Additional roles of fats (no pun intended) are to make foods more appetizing, provide a satiety value, and as the most concentrated form of energy. We have also discovered in recent years the essential roles that fats play in cellular membrane structure, in hormone synthesis, and prostagladin formation (a hormone-like group of compounds involved in a myriad of body functions). However, none of these activities is likely to be compromised by even low-fat diets; even the poorest Asiatic diet is 10% fat in content, and most "fat-free" diets in this country rarely get below 5%.

It is, therefore, most essential that we try to minimize our animal fat intake as well as lower the overall total consumption of fats. The unsaturated fats found in plants are more healthful than the saturated ones oozing from our excessive meat diet. For the active athlete the intake of fats must be further regulated. The major reason that fats have a satiety value is due to their slow transit time through the stomach and small intestine. This is an advantage if you are dieting, but a major disadvantage when active. You do not want needed blood shunted from exercising muscles to the gut in order to digest that burger and fries. Therefore, most athletes eat little or no fats while active, as well as restricting their intake just prior to endurance events. I personally do not eat any significant amount of fats within four or five hours of long bike rides or races.

PROTEINS

Proteins are compounds which contain nitrogen in addition to the carbon, hydrogen and oxygen (some also contain a trace of sulphur, phosphorus and other trace minerals). Protein comes from a Greek word with the root meaning "to come first." The etymology is apt indeed; proteins are the essential building materials for all living matter. They are needed to build new tissue, repair old tissue, as regulatory substances in salt and water balance, as precursors to hormones, vitamins, antibodies and enzymes—in addition to their energy-supplying role.

All proteins are not of equal nutritional value. Proteins are composed of amino acids—small nitrogen-containing molecules. Some amino acids can be synthesized by the human body; these are called "non-essential" amino acids. Other amino acids cannot be synthesized; these are known as "essential" amino acids. It is for this reason that a diet may contain quantitatively enough protein, but not qualitatively. In 1956 the Food and Agricultural Organization of the United Nations rated certain foods according to their amino acid content. Eggs were found to contain the best balance of "essential" amino acids, and were given a 100% rating. All other foods were rated in comparison to eggs. Thus, milk is 60%, fish and meat 70%, soybeans 69%, peanuts 34%, white flour 32%, corn 41%, rice 56%, and potato 34%. This is the basis for attempts to produce grains with higher levels of "essential" amino acids. A major breakthrough has been the development of a type of corn with a high lysine content (an "essential" amino acid usually found in small quantities in corn). This can raise corn's rating to 61%. Nevertheless, vegetarian diets must be constructed carefully in order to avoid problems involving low intake of "essential" amino acids.

A vegetarian diet which includes milk and cheese is unlikely to be poor in amino acids, but a strictly vegan diet (avoiding any animal source) can easily be grossly deficient. This has been seen in tragic proportions in the small group of young people who have adhered to the "Zen Macrobiotic Diet." This is an extremely dangerous diet; several deaths have been reported as a result of it. This is not meant to be a putdown of vegetarian diets; I think they have a lot to offer. Yet, they require some careful planning in order to avoid stupid, unhealthy results.

The other side of the coin is the question of how much protein is best suited for good health, and whether exercise alters this in any way. In 1881 Voit studied the diets of German workers, and concluded from their average protein consumption that 118 grams/day was a desirable level. This level is still quoted, but more careful studies have shown that this is greatly in excess of the actual human requirement. Current research would suggest that 25–45 grams/day would be a more appropriate intake. In fact, a recent article in *The Lancet* suggested that the current UN calculations for protein needs of the devastated drought-ridden African nations were over-estimated. It was suggested that very low levels of "essential" amino acid consumption are compatible with good health.

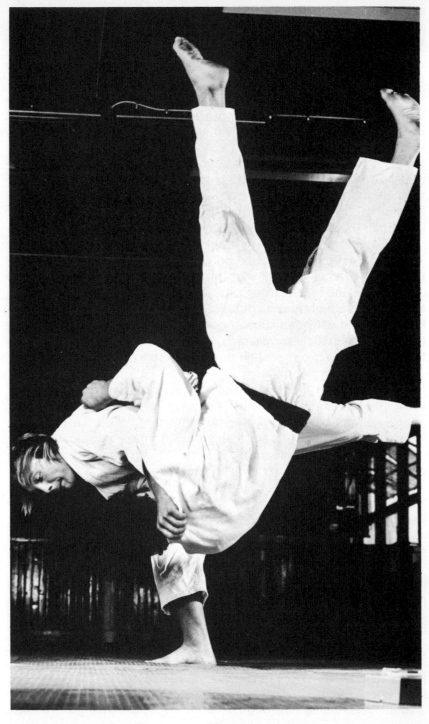

This may be challenged by the data pointing to protein deficiency as a major contributing factor in mental retardation and behavior problems in children, even in this country.

Athletes have also contended that because of their active muscle turnover, they require more protein. Wrestlers, weight-lifters and field competitors seem to endorse this theory more than other sportsmen. However, it is worth noting that not a single experiment (and dozens have been performed to test this hypothesis) has demonstrated the benefit of a high protein diet, either for developing muscle strength or endurance. In fact, recent studies indicate that high protein diets may be detrimental because of the resulting increase in bioactive amines which may actually depress brain and nerve functions. Finally, protein is usually linked to fat (especially in animal forms), and again the problem of slow transit through the digestive tract is a problem for the exercising individual.

VITAMINS

Although the history of vitamin research dates back to 1880 in Estonia where Lunin revealed that mice maintained on artificial protein, fat and carbohydrate died, the field is still entwined by fragmentary data and scores of unanswered questions. With the vitamin battle now taking on a quasi-religious tone it is almost impossible to discuss vitamins without irritating someone. Let me, therefore, confine my comments to the question of vitamin requirements in exercise, and what is known about excessive vitamin intake.

First, let me dismiss vitamins A and D. They are not involved in muscle, nerve, or cardiac physiology to any great degree. Unless you are on a very low fat diet it is nearly impossible to be deficient in these vitamins (they are added to many foods). Furthermore, large doses of both of these vitamins have proven serious toxic effects, even potentially lethal ones. Vitamin A toxicity may produce brain, liver or eye damage. Vitamin D in excess can cause serious kidney damage.

Vitamin C is a more difficult topic. There is no doubt that several recent studies have indicated Linus Pauling may be correct in his theory that megadoses of vitamin C (1–4 grams/day) will prevent or reduce the symptoms of common viral ailments, especially the cold. Some investigators have suggested that at those high

Brian Jacks throws Anguzo Parisi in a judo match in Great Britain. Explosive strength depends on a supply of muscle glycogen and metabolic efficiency that comes from eating "pure fuels" exclusively. (Tony Duffy Photo)

levels of ingestion vitamin C acts as an antihistamine rather than as a primary anti-viral agent.

Vitamin C in large doses is not without harm; it may cause kidney stones or nausea, and most disturbing is the recent report indicating that large doses of C block 40–60% of vitamin B_{12} in the gastrointestinal tract. If this proves to be consistently demonstrated, one would want to take vitamin C at times separated from meals as far as possible, especially in vegetarian diets where B_{12} is already at low levels. However, I confess that I am still a believer of the double-Nobel laureate's ideas, and supplement my diet with vitamin C.

The other fashionable vitamin is E. Here, there is not a shred of responsible scientific data to indicate that supplementation is beneficial. In experiments with vitamin E-free diets volunteers could not be rendered deficient in E after 16 months on the diet. No disease state in man is known to be improved by E ingestion. Perhaps most pertinent for our readers is the fact that several recent studies in this country and Europe have investigated the effect of E on athletes. Cyclists, runners, wrestlers and footballers have all been studied. There is not a shred of evidence that E supplements increased strength or endurance. In fact, two studies suggested it was detrimental in massive doses. Admittedly no toxic effect of E is known, but I suspect some American professor of medicine will make his name by describing a disease state resulting from excessive E intake. Just last year that occurred in the case of nicotinic acid.

The B vitamins are another matter altogether. Thiamine (B_1) is especially important to athletes. It is vitally linked to carbohydrate metabolism and especially lactic acid utilization. Thus, the high carbohydrate diet of many athletes requires more thiamine than the ordinary diet. This is in addition to the fact that most Americans are consuming borderline amounts of this vitamin. Repeated studies have demonstrated that low levels of thiamine are associated with irritability and lassitude. It has been called the "morale vitamin." Exercising athletes on moderately high carbohydrate diets require at least 2 mg/day. A recent study in the southern states revealed that 20% of school children consume less than one mg/day. There is no evidence that excessive thiamine is of any benefit, but many of us are thiamine deficient. Except for seeds, wheat germ and nuts, meat is the best source of thiamine. Vegetarian diets should routinely include yeast products, wheat germ or nuts.

Other B vitamins are less essential to the athlete. However, a few brief comments should be made. Riboflavin (B_2) is required in many processes involving cellular repair and growth. Diets with no milk products included are very likely to be riboflavin deficient. Milk supplies 45% of the riboflavin consumed in this country. Niacin (once known as B_5) is the pellagra-preventing factor. Deficiencies of this vitamin are most common in diets consisting of rice, corn and highly-milled flour.

A riboflavin-deficient diet will usually be a niacin-deficient one as well. Pyridoxine (B_6) is coupled closely to niacin and riboflavin. In the milling of white flour 75% of the B_6 content is lost. Wheat germ, nuts and yeast are, again, good sources of pyridoxine. None of the B complex has been shown to be beneficial in megadoses. There is a current controversy about these vitamins in psychiatric use, but this is not the place to consider this confusing and confused subject.

A special word of caution must be reiterated about vitamin B_{12}. There is none in yeast, the traditional source of B vitamins. Milk and its products are high in B_{12}, as are meats. However, this vitamin is not very stable; 40–90% of it is destroyed in the processing of evaporated milk. If you suspect that your diet is B_{12} deficient, you can supplement with B_{12} pills from microbial growth concentrates. B_{12} deficiency can cause a severe degeneration of the brain and spinal cord as well as an anemia. In fact, a mild anemia may plague a patient for many years before its cause is found. It was formerly felt that an unnecessary amount of B_{12} supplements were given by doctors for vague and non-specific complaints. However, with the increasing tendency toward more plant-oriented diets, B_{12} supplements should be re-examined.

MINERALS

The most essential minerals to fluid and salt balance are sodium, potassium and chloride. However, the aspects of water and salt balance are sufficiently complex that they cannot be adequately discussed in this type of survey. Let me turn, therefore, to the lesser minerals.

Calcium is essential for bone structure, blood coagulation and the rhythmic contraction of muscles (including the heart). Certain substances may bind calcium (oxalic acid in cocoa and phytic acid in cereals) or excessive fats may tie up calcium in the gut as "soaps." Yet, calcium deficiencies are not common in the US. The best sources of calcium are hard cheese, milk, green vegetables and fish bones. Probably the most important fact about calcium in regards to athletics is the fact that it competes with magnesium for absorption from the gastrointestinal tract.

Magnesium has been shown to be essential in preventing muscle cramps (especially in hot weather). I routinely try to eat nuts, soybeans or wheat germ in the hot cycling season. I absolutely avoid milk products during hot rides so that there is no blocking of magnesium absorption. Most American diets are not rich in magnesium, and athletes would do well to consciously seek higher intakes of this vital mineral. It causes diarrhea when taken in supplement forms, so dietary intake is preferable. With adequate magnesium in the diet, salt tablets are not necessary on even the hottest days.

Most readers realize that iron is the essential metal in hemoglobin (the oxygen-carrying pigment of the blood). Yet, it is not commonly recognized that a sizeable portion of the population suffers from iron deficiency. Recent surveys have indicated that 10–12% of American men are iron deficient, and more than 20% of women are. As I pointed out in a recent *Bike World* issue, recent research has demonstrated that women are capable of achieving maximum oxygen uptake levels comparable with those of men, if they are not iron deficient. I personally think that any female athlete still menstruating should supplement her diet with either ferrous sulfate or ferrous fumarate tablets.

Good food sources of iron include eggs, lean meat, nuts, dried fruits, whole grains, raisins and dark molasses. The athlete trying to push his oxygen uptake over 70 cannot afford to be even mildly anemic due to an iron-poor diet.

Zinc has enjoyed its spotlight of renewed interest since the early 1960's. Diets low in zinc and high in calcium or phylates (grains and beans) may lead to disorders of appetite and poor bone metabolism. Zinc is not plentiful in vegetables, but is abundant in meats. Zinc deficiencies are not common in this country, except in alcoholics. It is an essential element in insulin and enzymes catalyzing protein synthesis. No increased demand is created by exercise.

Other trace minerals include manganese, fluoride, selenium, chromium, nickel, tin, vanadium and silicon. The details of these metals' roles in nutrition are being investigated in many centers throughout the world. Any one of them may become an important topic as eating habits change, some foods become scarce, and additives and processing radically alter normal metabolic inter-relations.

I have tried to keep this article from sounding like "my" diet recommendations. I hope the information has been adequate so that each reader can construct his own diet knowledgeably. Yet, let me summarize by highlighting some of the factors which seem important to me as I read the nutritional literature:

● Carbohydrates are the best energy source while active, and carbohydrate-loading is endorsed by many athletes in preparing for long races.

● There is no evidence that increased levels of exercise require a high protein diet. Most American diets are probably excessive in protein content.

● The vitamin B complex is supplied in only marginal amounts in our diet. Active athletes would probably benefit from B supplementation.

● Vitamin E maintains its undisputed position as the modern day snake medicine—a fortune producer for its vendors and worthless for its faithful addicts.

● Vegetarian diets can be accepted by athletes, but they should be carefully planned in order to avoid deficiencies in essential amino acids, B_{12}, riboflavin and zinc.

● Milk and milk products should not be consumed just before, during, or just after strenuous exercise in hot weather in order that the calcium of these compounds not interfere with magnesium uptake.

● Most women athletes should take supplemental iron if they wish to enjoy their fullest potential as athletes.

● The current intense interest in nutritional research will undoubtedly bring many other important metabolic facts to sports medicine in the very near future.

LEGACY OF SUPERSTITION

Athletics is full of old wives' tales. A pitcher won't change caps 'til the end of the season—bad luck, you know. A marathon runner doesn't shave on race day—makes him feel mean and "run faster." A bike racer shines every last screw on his bike—intimidates his opposition.

Nowhere is superstition more flagrantly and unquestioningly adhered to by thousands of athletes who never bothered to look twice than in diet. Let's take a look at a few time-hallowed principles of the way athletes do or don't eat. You'll find more information on each of these points as you read further in *Food for Fitness*.

Every body needs milk. Not so. In the first place, as Dr. Ralph Bircher shows in his review of the research, excess protein is not only unnecessary but may be toxic. Secondly, the amino acid balance of cow's milk is quite different from that required for optimal human nutrition—goat's milk is much closer to the ideal. Last but not least, there are millions of people whose stomachs simply do not produce the enzymes necessary to digest milk properly.

Every body needs bread. Another myth. It's been found that, like milk, millions of people have trouble with wheat proteins. Wheat digestion is ticklish business—its combination of starch and protein demands enzyme production by the stomach for the breakdown of each of these elements—at the same time. Many stomachs haven't learned this trick. This is true of many racial groups for whom wheat has not been the staple grain—orientals and blacks, for example.

Steak for breakfast is best on game day. Steak may sit in your stomach for as long as four hours before even entering the intestinal tract. Its stressful metabolic toxins such as urea give the body's eliminative systems an extra chore on a day when they'll already have extra work to do—getting rid of the byproducts of exercise stresses. The proteins of meat are only very slowly converted to sugars for energy. Steak has very little usefulness as a pre-event food.

Candy bars give you a lift. Yes, they do—and they let you down hard. This is thoroughly discussed in the chapter on harmful foods. The entire "quick energy" myth is a giant rip-off invented by the food industry that led you to eat things that make you feel sluggish in the first place. Dextrose pills, tea loaded with sugar, athletic drinks and even nature's own honey all have their limits. The further from nature these products are, the more drastic their limitations.

Plain white sugar and dextrose pills produce "reactive hypoglycemia"—your blood sugar rises quickly, making you feel great for awhile, then the body's balance-preserving mechanisms react to send insulin into the bloodstream. Bang—late in the game you don't feel so hot anymore.

Sugars in milder concentration produce a less startled reaction by the body and are better for pre-event and mid-event use. Orange

Tom Dooley and Steve Lansing race walk at 5000 meters—salt pills, protein powders, candy bars and steak, all items from dietary mythology, have no positive effect on such races. (John Marconi)

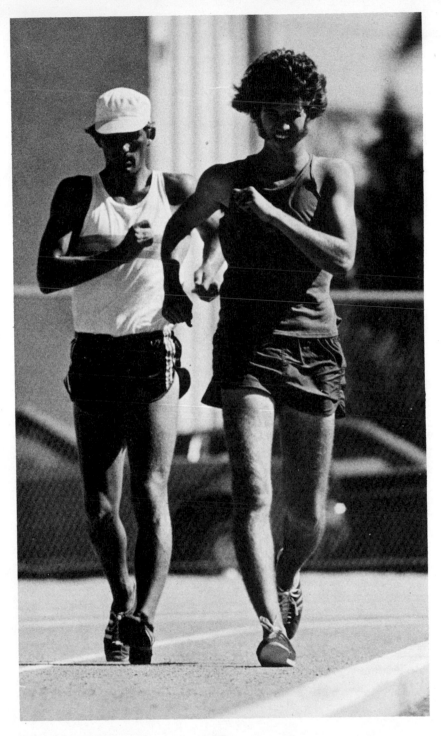

juice, E.R.G. and other dilute sources are safer and provide usable sources of minerals, vitamins and enzymes also lost in competition.

Wheat germ and honey are the ideal athlete's food. You can't eat trash all day long and gobble wheat germ and honey, expecting some chemical miracle to save you from your transgressions of natural law. If we make one point in this book we hope that it will be this: there are no dietary wonders—there are only the potentially wonderful effects of following fixed natural laws.

Wheat germ is great food, if you can get it fresh—often it goes rancid on the grocer's shelf. If you have stomach trouble with wheat germ, try the health food store for a fresh supply. If you still have problems, you may be one of those whose stomach can't handle the enzyme problems of digesting wheat.

Wheat germ and honey is a lousy food combination. The problem is that each interferes with the digestion of the other. Honey when eaten with other foods is held up in the stomach, instead of passing as it normally would, straight into the intestine. It starts to ferment in the stomach and this condition almost guarantees acid fermentation. Honey has an inhibiting effect on the secretion of digestive juices in the stomach, making digestion of the wheat germ less than optimal.

Protein pills build muscles and energy. Protein pills build muscular bank balances for those who sell them. They're a testimonial to the nutritional ignorance of those who buy them. As Ralph Bircher points out in his article, daily protein requirements even for athletes are much lower than previously suspected. Excess protein may actually be poisonous, according to Bircher's summary of protein research. Protein pills often are made of heated soya and other proteins. Heating destroys all the enzymes and a good deal of the amino acid structure of proteins, making them less useful for the body and creating a stress for the body's eliminative organs. Soy beans cost less than 20 cents a pound in bulk. Protein pills, with perhaps egg or other proteins thrown in, cost as much as a dollar a pound and more. You figure it out.

Even 100% natural, unheated, egg-protein-based protein pills or powders would be truly an impractical source of amino acids for a person concerned with economy as well as health. They are a play upon our national conviction that pills hold answers to problems.

Protein gives you a quick lift before an event. Protein is the slowest-digesting food of all, and is ranked fourth behind fruit sugars, starchy foods and fats as a source of glucose for the working muscles.

A good hot meal gives you energy for competition. Cooking robs food of an enormous amount of its value, and converts it into a devitalizing, fermenting dietary nightmare. The heat of cooking is quickly lost—long before the food reaches the point in the intestinal tract at which its available carbohydrates are absorbed into the bloodstream and turned into energy and heat.

Eat every day from the "four basic food groups." The basic groups referred to in this slogan are milk and dairy products, meat, bread and cereals, and fruit and vegetables. As you'll learn in *Food for Fitness,* two of these "essential" food groups are indigestible by millions of individuals with wheat or milk intolerances. Meat is an expensive, unecological source of protein, inferior because of the toxic byproducts of its digestion. On the basis of the physiology of the human digestive tract, it is not even a natural food for man. Carnivores have shorter digestive tubes, corresponding to meat's quick rate of decomposition. By this criterion man is a fruit-eater. Meat begins to rot, producing a breeding ground for harmful bacteria, before it leaves the human body. Researchers are beginning to attribute much cancer of the intestines and colon to meat-eating.

You need salt pills in hot weather. Rommel's troops fought in the hot North African desert in good health without any table salt at all. Marathoners have recently found that an otherwise balanced but completely salt-free diet makes them much *better,* rather than worse, hot-weather runners. Scientists testing athletes and field workers have found that the main electrolyte lost in sweat during competition is not the sodium of salt, but magnesium and potassium, for which the best sources are fruit and vegetables.

One beer can't hurt on a hot day. One beer can lower your heat tolerance for as long as three days.

Bananas are great for racing cyclists. In a recent *Bike World* survey of 60 top US racing cyclists it was found that most ate this much-lauded fruit during races. Bananas are a good source of fruit sugars, vitamins and minerals—but nothing is digested as quickly as liquids. The extra work of digesting solid food can only hinder performance and perhaps some of the best racing cyclists have intuitively realized this, replacing their bananas with fluid energy sources.

Carbohydrate loading means you can really go to town on bread and other starches. One distance runner using this five-day pre-event diet (described elsewhere in *Food for Fitness*) ate several loaves of bread at a sitting on one of his high-carbo days, felt chest pains, and was subsequently advised by his physician to stay completely out of training and competition for an extended period because of resultant irregularities in his heart rhythms. Carbohydrate loading is not a license. Overeating at *any* time is counterproductive—your liver's glycogen storage capacity is a fixed quantity and eating beyond the point where you no longer feel hungry is perfectly useless.

Diet is the big compensator. There are no diet miracles, just as there are no dope miracles. Good diet is helpful—essential—but it is only as good as your training and heredity, as far as competitive results go. For basic health and feeling good, it's indispensable.

Athletes need a lot more vitamins. This is quite true, as several authors in *Food for Fitness* point out. But the body can use effectively only a fixed quantity of each vitamin, which varies between individuals, and all vitamins must be present in combination with balanced amounts of minerals, trace elements and other nutritional substances. The safest way to provide an optimally harmonious balance is by improving the way you eat vitamins as they come out of the ground—not out of a jar. The human race grew up in a symbiotic relationship with nature, and the proper balance of nutritional elements, including vitamins, is found in natural foods.

After medical researchers found runners' bodies used larger than normal amounts of vitamins C and E and magnesium, there was a rash of pill-popping among marathoners. Those whose diet had previously been adequate experienced no change whatsoever in performance. Those who'd been eating imbalanced diets deficient in one of the vitamins experienced "miraculous" performance increases. The superstitious continue to gulp their miracle pills.

Drinks are bad before, during or after a workout. Believe it or not, there are still track coaches who'll have their athletes run long sessions of repeat intervals on a hot day without liquid intake. The article on drinks in *Food for Fitness* should drown this ancient wisdom forever.

All athletes need a high carbohydrate diet for energy. Like most generalizations, this is a half-truth. Athletes obviously need a lot of energy from foods. The source which the body can use most easily is fruit, followed in order of digestive ease by starchy carbohydrates like whole grain and cereal products and potatoes. Fruit is preferred for its easy digestibility and abundant content of the enzymes, minerals and vitamins specifically required for physical performance.

Athletes are extremely sensitive to changes in their health and performance capacity, so it's natural that they should be attracted to the promise of quick and easy improvements through eating. The more intelligent, however, will look twice at the sloganized "wisdom" that has long ruled the training table. *Food for Fitness* has been written for athletes who want to take a closer look.

SOMETHING FOR EVERYONE

There are several ideas behind this chart. Its most obvious purpose is to help you locate the topics in *Food for Fitness* that apply to your particular sport. Another is to surprise you. Many findings in this book clash with old ideas about athletic diet, and the chart reflects this. The reason we were able to make revolutionary judgments in ranking the importance of different diet practices is that the research is there to back us up.

Bobby Fischer may have been chosen Sportsman of the Year but you won't find chess listed here. Our standard for selecting sports was that performance of the heart-lung system and/or musculature must be involved. In borderline cases like "fishing" we considered the extreme situation: ocean fishing with its extended exertions. Target shooting, for example, was dropped. Even though hand-eye coordination is a physical performance factor in that sport which could be influenced by diet, the effort is so slight and so intermittent as to make diet's influence marginal at best. Our letter grades were defined like this:

A Indispensable. When the diet factor in question is neglected, performance inevitably suffers greatly.

B Important. In some cases, can be neglected without loss of health, but must be considered for optimal results.

C Helpful. Advisable for maintenance of health, general condition or competitive results, as a normal adjunct to training or competition.

D Occasionally useful. Not a constant factor, but in some cases can affect performance if used in preparing for or during competition, or for recovery.

F Not a factor. Will not improve performance if general diet is adequate.

X Harmful.

Carbo-loading's no good for bowling? Wouldn't it be better for a bowler to go to the line with four times as much stored glycogen in his liver? Frankly, no. First, carbo-loading only makes a difference in continuous hard exercise of at least an hour and a half duration. And it shouldn't be abused; as we've pointed out elsewhere in *Food for Fitness,* carbo-loading is an insult to the body's stress adaptation mechanisms, and the body won't take much insulting without being seriously weakened somewhere.

General diet got high grades. Otto Brucker makes the irrefutable point that what's good for health is good for performance. Who can argue with that? A vitamin A deficiency will adversely affect performance in archery, for example, and if you get too little vitamin B_1 you'll feel like climbing in your golf bag and curling up for about 10 years' sleep.

"But I *like* to eat solid foods during a long bicycle race," you say. Well and good, but the reason we ranked this practice below drinking is that digesting solid food robs performance energy from from the working muscles, while drinking does so to a much less severe extent. It's your choice—we're not the final authority, only reviewers of the available research findings.

To back up our gradings on "general diet," we drew on information throughout *Food for Fitness.* We also looked at the degree of hard physical work demanded in a sport: the more strenuous the sport, the more importance we gave general diet. Our prime reference for doing this was Dr. Otto Brucker's direct correlation of performance and basic health.

The pre-event and mid-event drink evaluations are based to some extent on little-known research findings. You'll be able to read all about this in the article on drinks.

In rating solid food consumption, we were concerned with two essential points. First was the fact that eating during strenuous physical exercise makes the body do an extra load of "digestive work." As physiologists have pointed out, this is not a small matter—to push food through 30 feet of tubing is hard physical labor, and the effects on performance are definite and significant. "If you can go without eating, you're better off doing so," was our criterion. The second matter concerns length of the exercise period. Mountain climbing and backpacking can be carried on for months, and obviously solid food is going to be necessary on a Mt. Everest expedition.

Carbo-loading is effective, but controversial. For those readers who've never heard of it, carbohydrate loading is a five-day diet and exercise plan which results in an increase of as much as 400% in the liver's glycogen stores. You can get the details in the article on pre-event nutrition. Carbo-loading is used mainly by long-distance athletes like marathoners and bike racers. In events lasting less than 1½ hours it's practically a waste of time—it takes that long for the normal glycogen supplies to run out during hard endurance-paced exercise, and the special five-day diet only makes a difference at the beyond-an-hour-and-a-half level. Slightly increasing your fruit and natural grain intake for a couple of days before a race or game will "top up" your liver's glycogen without the need for a five-day routine.

Carbohydrate loading is stressful, and shouldn't be taken lightly. Several warnings are contained with the article on carbo-loading in *Food for Fitness,* but a good general principle is to view this practice as an unabashed exploitation to the body's stress reactions, and thus an unusual wear-and-tear on your performing metabolism.

Weight loss is obviously advantageous in some sports—long distance running, bicycle racing, and yet it was tricky to apply the grading system for this category. What's the starting point? If you're recovering from severe disease and in emaciated condition, weight loss may be deadly, even though your goal is to be a "skinny marathoner." If your weight is all "eaten-on" fat and you have trouble moving fast, weight gain may not help your football career. In both these cases we took the conservative line and advised that weight loss "may be helpful." For long distance running, we "X-rated" weight gain, again ignoring extremes and upholding the general principle that for most people in distance running, it will be advantageous and safe to lose some weight. Marathon runners' optimal weights often lie up to 20% under insurance company "normal" standards, and even runners with large training pensums must often do "dietary work" to get down to best racing levels.

One general principle emerges from the chart, and it's one that you'll find repeated throughout the book. Maximum performance is impossible with a body in less than optimal health. "I eat everything, and don't suffer," is the standard retort of those who judge diet's effects without submitting them to the test of experimentation. Let the research and results speak for themselves.

Requirements for Sports

	GENERAL DIET	PRE-EVENT DRINKS	MID-EVENT DRINKS	PRE-EVENT FOOD	MID-EVENT FOOD	CARBO-LOADING	WEIGHT LOSS	WEIGHT GAIN
Alpine skiing	B	D	D	C	F	F	F	F
Archery	C	F	D	D	F	F	D	F
Auto Racing	B	C	C	C	D	D	D	X
Backpacking	C	D	C	D	C	F	F	X
Badminton	C	F	D	D	F	F	D	F
Baseball	B	C	C	C	F	F	D	X
Basketball	A	A	A	A	X	C	F	X
Bicycling	B	B	C	B	D	D	F	X
Boating	C	D	D	D	X	F	D	F
Bobsledding	C	F	F	D	F	F	D	X
Bowling	C	F	D	D	D	F	D	F
Boxing	A	A	B	A	X	D	D	D
Canoeing	B	C	C	D	D	F	F	X
Cricket	C	F	D	D	F	F	F	F
Cross-Country Skiing	B	B	D	C	D	D	D	F
Curling	C	F	D	D	D	F	F	F
Diving	C	D	F	D	X	F	F	F
Dog Packing	C	D	C	D	D	F	D	F
Dog Sled Racing	B	C	B	B	D	C	D	X
Equestrian	C	D	D	D	F	F	F	X
Fencing	C	D	D	D	F	F	D	F
Field Hockey	B	C	B	B	X	D	F	D
Figure Skating	B	D	D	D	F	F	F	F
Fishing	C	F	D	D	C	F	F	F
Football	A	A	A	A	X	D	D	D
Golf	C	F	D	D	D	F	F	F
Gymnastics	A	C	C	D	F	F	D	X
Handball	B	C	C	B	X	D	F	F

	GENERAL DIET	PRE-EVENT DRINKS	MID-EVENT DRINKS	PRE-EVENT FOOD	MID-EVENT FOOD	CARBO-LOADING	WEIGHT LOSS	WEIGHT GAIN
Hang Gliding	C	F	F	D	F	F	F	X
Hiking	C	D	C	D	C	F	F	F
Ice Hockey	A	C	C	C	F	F	F	D
Jogging	C	D	F	D	F	F	D	X
Judo	C	D	D	D	X	F	F	F
Karate	C	D	D	D	X	F	F	F
Kayaking	C	C	D	D	X	F	F	F
Lacrosse	B	C	C	C	F	F	F	D
Marathon Running	A	A	A	A	D	C	D	X
Martial Arts	C	D	D	D	X	F	F	F
Middle Distance Running	B	C	F	C	X	D	D	F
Modern Pentathlon	C	C	C	B	X	D	D	F
Motorcycling	C	D	C	D	F	F	F	F
Mountain Climbing	B	C	C	B	C	F	D	X
Orienteering	B	C	C	C	F	D	D	F
Paddleball	B	C	C	C	X	D	F	F
Parachuting	C	F	F	D	F	F	F	F
Race Walking	B	C	C	C	D	D	D	F
Rafting	C	C	D	D	X	F	F	F
Raquetball	B	C	C	C	X	D	D	F
Rock Climbing	B	C	C	D	D	F	D	X
Roller Skating	C	F	D	D	D	F	F	F
Rowing	B	D	C	C	X	D	F	F
Rugby	A	B	C	B	F	D	D	D
Sailing	C	C	D	C	X	F	F	F
Scuba Diving	B	D	F	C	X	F	F	F
Skin Diving	B	D	F	C	X	F	F	F
Snowshoeing	A	B	C	B	D	D	F	X
Soccer	A	A	A	A	X	D	D	D
Softball	C	D	D	D	F	F	F	F
Speed Skating	A	C	F	C	F	F	D	X
Sprinting	B	D	F	C	X	F	D	X
Squash	B	C	D	C	X	D	D	D

	GENERAL DIET	PRE-EVENTS DRINKS	MID-EVENT DRINKS	PRE-EVENT FOOD	MID-EVENT FOOD	CARBO-LOADING	WEIGHT LOSS	WEIGHT GAIN
Surfing	C	D	F	C	X	F	F	F
Swimming	B	D	F	C	X	F	F	F
Synchronized Swimming	C	D	F	D	X	F	F	F
Table Tennis	C	F	D	D	F	F	F	F
Tennis	B	C	D	C	D	D	D	F
Track & Field (Field)	B	C	F	C	X	D	D	D
Ultra-Distance Running	A	A	A	A	D	C	D	X
Volleyball	B	C	D	C	F	F	F	F
Water Polo	B	D	F	C	X	F	F	F
Water Skiing	C	D	F	D	X	F	F	F
Weightlifting	A	B	F	C	F	D	D	D
Wrestling	A	B	F	C	F	D	D	F
Yachting	C	D	D	C	X	F	F	F
Yoga	B	F	F	D	F	F	F	F

2

The Life of Foods

"The athlete is attempting to maximize performance, and he realizes that any disturbance in the physical system will hinder him." Nutrition researcher Dr. Otto Brucker sets the theme for this chapter. Athletes must learn to fuel their bodies with the care that a proud sports car owner lavishes on his machine. A high performance engine demands special fuels of a certain high octane rating. No competent race driver would even think of competing without having carefully checked to make sure his car will be fueled properly before and during the event. Applying the same logic to the athlete's finely-tuned body-machine, it's essential for optimal performance to supply only the very highest quality fuels via food and drink, before and during competition.

"So why not just save the high octane stuff for race day, and not worry about it so much the rest of the time?" This is a common train of thought among athletes: "It's fanatical and tiresome to worry about diet all the time, and probably not all that necessary in any case."

A grand prix car generally sits in the garage between races or practice drives. It's given the very best by way of tuneups and cleaning. Not so the athlete's—or anybody's—body. It "races" every day. And far more important, it is given the extra task of reconstructing itself and improving upon its own efficiency. When parts in a race car engine wear out, they're simply replaced and the engine works as well as when it was new. Human parts are harder to replace. Nerves, kidneys, liver, intestines and other organs that have become worn and sludged from improper fueling are first of all inefficient; and in the cases where it's not too late, cleaning them out and getting them to run smoothly still takes

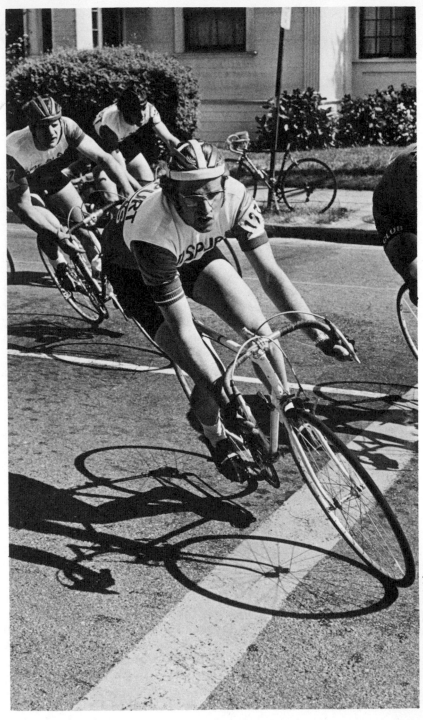

time—you can't just pop in a new kidney and roar out on the road again. The fuels for rebuilding are just as important as those for racing.

In this chapter you'll learn what "clean fuels" for the body are—how to save your body the extra work of handling inefficient fuels and turn that saved energy into increased athletic performance. You'll also find out which foods are optimal for the body's "other work" which isn't directly involved with energy for competition: the constant daily chore of rebuilding and improving the tissue of which the body is made. Putting high octane fuel in a Model T is useless. The body—an energy-conversion machine—is itself refined and made more efficient by proper food—the Model T body may become a Ferrari with training, proper diet and other hygienic factors.

We can't remind you often enough: it may seem a little complicated at times, but it's not. A good diet is quite simple. But to live simply in the midst of complexity is not easy. It takes long-range thinking—a righteous desire to have the best that one's body can deliver, and a patient willingness to keep on experimenting and learning until results come.

BASIC BODILY UPKEEP

by Dr. Otto Brucker

Anyone who enters athletics announces indirectly that he is not interested in neglecting his body. The athlete is attempting to maximize performance, and he realizes that any disturbance in the physical system will hinder him. His body's complicated metabolic system has to operate at best efficiency, and a basic condition for this is fulfilling nutritional needs.

However, the growing number of nutritionally-caused diseases and the high percentage of people afflicted indicates that the basic nutritional needs of the society are not being adequately met.

What is especially dangerous for the athlete is the widespread concept that he can prevent these diseases simply by exercising. This is not to say exercise is not important in the maintenance of health. But the athlete should keep the following firmly in mind: a man can stay healthy with proper nutrition but without sufficient movement; he *cannot* remain healthy on any amount of exercise if essential nutritional elements are lacking.

The ravages of modern nutrition cannot be prevented or softened by any kind of athletic activity. Despite the obvious physical benefits of exercise, it is clear that this activity cannot make up for the lack of essential metabolic substances. The reverse is more often the case. The more intense the physical movement, the more necessary is a sufficient supply of vital substances.

Just what constitutes a "sufficient supply of vital substances" is still open to some question. But a new body of nutritional research is currently replacing (or at least modifying) conventional medical thinking on this subject. Since these new findings have long since passed the stage of theory and have the test of practical application behind them, it seems negligent to continue quoting older nutritional theses. The most important matters in this "new nutrition" only become clear when contrasted with old theories (which, though outdated, still influence thinking today).

Old nutritional theory assumed that a supply of the three basic nutritional elements—protein, fat and carbohydrates—along with certain minerals was sufficient for health. These were supposed to give 2000–4000 calories a day. Measurement in terms of caloric content is a mark of old nutrition—not even the discovery of vitamins changed anything in this basic principle. Vitamins were merely added to the existing list of recommendations.

New nutritionists have discovered that the three basic substances, certain minerals and the classic vitamins are in no way enough to maintain health and performance capacity. Countless other substances are required. They are called "vital substances." These include not only the generally recognized vitamins and minerals, but also minerals present in the tiniest amounts ("trace elements"), a large group of enzymes, polyunsaturated fatty acids, and aromatic substances. Some of these are necessary for good health; others *must* be present for life itself to go on.

The common cause of performance lags and nutritionally associated diseases lies in the incorrect concepts of older nutritional theory: an over-emphasis on nutritional concentrates (isolated elements in the diet), and an underestimation of total nutritional needs.

Injury to health comes mainly from manufactured nutritional products. These are marked by a lack of vital substances that are essential. The more concentrated the substance is, the fewer vital elements it will contain and the more harmful it will be.

In old nutritional theory, the worth of a diet was measured by its caloric content. In the new order of things, nutrition is based on the diet's vitality. The more food is left to nature, the more alive it is; the less natural, the less lifelike. The scale extends from completely lifeless industrial preparations such as white sugar, to conserved and heated nutrients, to foods in their natural state.

Nutritional researcher Kollath set up a scientifically exact order of preference in his book *The Order of Our Nutrition*—in descending order of vitality: (1) completely natural; (2) fermentatively altered; (3) mechanically altered; (4) heated; (5) conserved; (6) artificially concentrated.

The two main representatives of isolated nutritional concentrates with insufficient vital substances are (1) *white sugar*, and (2) *refined flours*. Their danger is considerably greater than is generally recognized, and is based on the following three points:

- *They are practically void of vital substances*
- *They are eaten daily in large amounts by modern man*
- *Their harmfulness is still unknown by most people*

The growing number of industrially altered fats also contributes to ill health. These include margarines and oil products made by chemical processes. Other manufactured dietary items are less dangerous because of their low consumption.

Nutrients that contain no vital substances can be called "dead foods." In this sense, Kollath distinguishes between food and nutritional concentrates. Kollath says these concentrates can no longer be considered "food" because they lack certain *essential elements necessary to support life and health*. "Food" is *alive*, because it contains all substances necessary for life and health.

The "industrial" sugars (white sugar, "raw" sugar, brown sugar, etc.) cause a chain reaction of harm. Not only do they lack vital substances; they also act as vitamin thieves because they require vitamins (particularly B vitamins) for their digestion. In addition, these sugars interfere with enzyme activities *central to the production of energy in athletics*.

It is misleading to say that eating isolated sugars increases energy. In fact, it *requires* great energy just to assimilate these products. Eating these sugars drains away vital substances while adding none; it disturbs enzyme functions and in the end increases strength and energy levels not at all.

Eating isolated sugar is damaging in yet another way—because of its quick assimilation. Pure sugar, especially dextrose (glucose), passes quickly through the intestinal walls into the bloodstream. This is dangerously portrayed as advantageous and desirable, based on old nutritional theory. In truth, it has a negative effect. The immediate rise in blood sugar level is followed by a dramatic drop to levels below norm. (This is called a "hypoglycemic" state.) If the athlete tries to boost himself back up with further sugar intake he creates an even greater imbalance in his blood sugar level.

Athletes should keep in mind that proper metabolism can take place *only* when all the necessary vital substances are delivered, in balanced relationships. This is true of sugar consumption, and also of eating harmful grain products such as white flour.

Kollath was one of those responsible for the discovery of vital substances. He first succeeded in causing diseases in animals by withholding certain of these nutrients.

Czech scientist Bernasek has gone further with Kollath's experiments. Bernasek has shown that a still larger number of unidentified vitamins exist. He fed rats a purely synthetic diet that contained all previously known vital substances necessary for maintaining life and health. Diseases nevertheless occurred.

The most remarkable part of these experiments was that pathological changes in organs were found in the first generation only to a limited degree. But they appeared more and more acutely from generation to generation. Beyond the fifth generation there was no further reproduction.

An equally important result of these tests was that all the damage was preventable by feeding whole grains.

These observations have a further striking parallel in human beings, who are now in the third and fourth generation of *not* eating whole grain products. The American diet resembles that of the rat insofar as carbohydrates consist predominantly of pure starch and sugar preparations; fats consist of margarines and chemically extracted oils; and proteins are denatured by heating processes. The "inexplicable" degenerative phenomena in man— especially in the nervous system—have a striking similarity with the pathological findings in rats encountered during Bernasek's experiments.

New nutritionists have uncovered a number of other important facts of great practical significance. The two leading ones are:

- *Vegetable proteins are just as valuable as animal proteins.*
- *Heating contributes to the destruction of proteins.*

Researchers Kollath and Bernasek also made key discoveries in protein. When protein substances were heated to a maximum

These hardy souls have just swum San Francisco's Golden Gate. The carbohydrate and fat requirements for feats like this need little comment. (Jerry Hawryluk Photo)

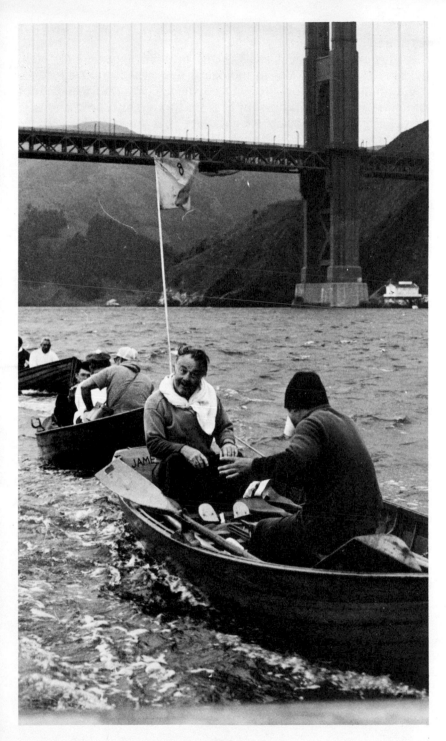

of 90°F, the laboratory rats lived normally. But when the heat was doubled, they died.

By purely chemical analysis the proteins appeared to retain the same properties. Yet in biological tests, the heated substance would no longer support life. The conclusion was that man cannot obtain an optimal protein supply from thoroughly cooked muscle meats, as was previously taught, but that uncooked vegetable nutrients supplemented with whole grains and cereals can do this. (Milk proteins likewise suffer severe damage from cooking and pasteurization processes.)

To summarize—it is clear that there is no important difference between the diet necessary for optimal health and the diet necessary for best performance in athletics. Although it is not possible in this short article to give details of a modern full-value diet, I can list general guidelines.

● The diet should consist, as much as possible, only of full-valued foods. I advise complete avoidance of manufactured nutrients. This means renouncing refined flour and sugar, and chemically-extracted fats.

● Take fruits and vegetables in raw form. The greater the share of raw products, the greater will be a person's performance capacity.

● Fill the protein needs with nuts, soy beans, whole grains and cereals, without relying on muscle meats.

● Drink only raw (unpasteurized) milk.

● Use only butter, cream and cold-pressed oils to fill fat needs.

It is important to recognize that health and performance capacity rest on several pillars. No single one contributes sufficiently without the others. Mastery of life's problems through harmony in the mental-spiritual realm is just as meaningful as whole-value natural nutrition, sufficient physical movement and abstention from enjoyable poisons. Only by a meaningful union of all factors can a person truly live.

FOOD KILLERS, KILLER FOODS

This chapter will repeat some of the ideas mentioned elsewhere, but this is the place where we'll go into food dangers in depth. For instance, Ralph Bircher makes some of the same general points about protein, and so does Otto Brucker. But many of the extra facts we gathered from a wide variety of sources will add to the reader's mental arsenal against ignorant eating habits.

CHEMICALS AND ADDITIVES

What's specifically wrong with additives? James Turner, author of *The Chemical Feast*, a brilliant exposé of the Food and Drug Administration, quotes researchers who consider food additive practices a "mutagenic time bomb." What this means in laymen's language is that certain of the chemicals now widely used in our industry-prepared foods can change human genetic structure—irreversibly. And the effects can't be cancelled out by switching to a chemical-free diet: it's a one-way street.

One of the great hygienists, J.H. Tilden, M.D., pointed out that toxin (poisonous substance) "is a by-product as constant and necessary as life itself. When the organism is normal, it is produced and eliminated as fast as produced." It's when we overload the body with chemicals it can't eliminate, or with too much toxin-producing foods, that we run into trouble. The result is "diseases of elimination": poisons are secreted from the body in mucus in the common cold, as pimples, and so on. And major organs of elimination like the liver and kidneys break down under the strain of too much work. Other parts of the body are similarly damaged by uneliminated poisons.

It would be impossible for us to run down the huge list of chemicals being added to our foods. All we can do is refer you to the bibliography and, on the basis of our own reading, say that you're better off avoiding *all* chemical additives. How to do it? You can switch to foods as close to their natural state as possible—raw fruits and vegetables, unprocessed whole wheat flour, whole grains and cereals, real eggs, etc. It's not uncommon for farmers to dump 200 pounds or more of chemicals on each acre of crops per season—so we're not talking about "trace amounts." It was estimated in 1970 that every average eater was consuming over five pounds of chemical additives a year. That gray powder on your grapes, plums, etc. probably contains far more bug killer and disease preventive than good old farm dust. Some commercial pesticides are so potent that a single drop of the pure active principle placed on your skin would kill you. As a good general reference we can mention Michael F. Jacobson's *Eater's Digest: The Consumer's Factbook of Food Additives* (Doubleday).

WHITE SUGAR

John Yudkin, M.D. is a famous British physician, biochemist and researcher who spent years studying the evils of sugar. Yudkin's work is extremely pertinent for the athlete, who's often tempted to get quick energy from candy bars, sugar drinks, etc. Before taking a look at what Yudkin learned in his research lab about the health dangers of white sugar, let's take a look at a phenomenon most athletes have either heard of or personally experienced—"sugar crash."

If you don't eat any sugar before a game or race, and your diet is otherwise adequate, you'll perform with a good supply of energy until all your liver's glycogen stores have been converted to glucose and delivered to the cells. During the event your body will also be converting a small percentage of stored fats into glucose and using this as a supplementary source of energy. You'll also be using mineral salts—mostly potassium, magnesium and sodium—and the enzymes involved in the energy conversion processes.

What happens when there's no more stored glycogen? If you have trained frequently on a low-carbohydrate diet or even fasted while doing endurance exercise, you may have taught your body to switch smoothly to burning stored fats as its energy source. Ernst van Aaken, M.D., a famous German trainer of marathon runners, claims this has been tested by his own athletes, including former 2000-meter world record holder and Olympic silver medalist Harald Norpoth.

If you *haven't* trained your body to convert to fats, using the "low burner" so to speak—and few athletes have—you're going to "crash" as your glycogen supplies disappear. If you've been doing endurance work for many years your liver will have a greater glycogen storage capacity than if you've just begun, and if you've "carbohydrate loaded" as described elsewhere in this book, you'll likewise have an extra margin of glycogen. But face it—this is only a small bonus and in a long race or game, sooner or later you'll have to eat or drink.

The best choice, of course, is to teach your body to go longer *before* entering a long event, given normal eating and drinking required by a long event. That's what training's all about, isn't it—to get the body ready to perform *naturally* what it's capable of doing, within natural limits. But if you believe in achieving ends by any means, you'll want to enter that long race prepared or not. So, you cautiously start eating well in advance of the point at which on the basis of your training experience you know you'll pass the limits of your trained condition. Or, you start swigging something like E.R.G.

You can feel the crash coming. The brain reacts with depression and reduced confidence when its glucose starts to run out. By this time it may be too late for preventive measures, though, so it's best to test your limits in training and calculate in advance when to start eating or drinking.

Many athletes have found it's better to drink all through a race or game at regular intervals—say every 10 miles in a bicycle race—than to start guzzling late in the event, which can cause stomach upset.

You can't run a 26-mile marathon on E.R.G. and a prayer. Not only would it prove nothing except that you're very good at drinking: it just doesn't work. You have to train your heart, lungs and energy-conversion systems to work that long.

"Sugar crash" means something else, too. You may decide it's safe to drink your electrolyte replacement or eat before your race, then take nothing along during the event. If you're a distance runner, for instance, and the race is considerably longer than you have prepared for in training, your "extra boost" will backfire. When the crash comes, it's going to be of epic proportions. Dr. Yudkin explains it like this: "A more than normally rapid absorpsorption of a great deal of glucose occurs if a lot of sugar is consumed . . . There is then a rapid rise of blood glucose, and an excessive amount of insulin is secreted. Because of this, the subsequent fall of blood glucose is excessive, the level becomes abnormally low, and if it is low enough symptoms of hypoglycemia will appear." Hypoglycemia is the crash—but with a vengeance.

Yudkin's research indicates it might not be wise to take sugar every day during normal training. "There is some evidence, too, that continued high intake of sugar can, at least for a time, result in an increased sensitivity of the pancreas, so that it responds more readily still by an increased secretion of insulin, and hypoglycemia becomes even more likely."

If you have the crash first and then take more E.R.G., you may limp over the finish line but the crowds will have gone home.

It takes a while for the new supplies of glucose and electrolytes to go to work; and even then, further complications of stomach upset and other unknown factors make it unlikely you'll return to before-crash efficiency. At least, this has been the experience of many distance runners and racing cyclists.

E.R.G. and the other commercial sports drinks contain glucose, not ordinary white sugar (sucrose). Yudkin says the difference is considerable, since glucose is the final energy-producing fuel of the cells, while many of white sugar's bad effects are the result of harmful processes involved in its digestion.

Even glucose should be used sparingly. Drs. F.C. Dohan and F.D.W. Lukens of the George S. Cox Medical Research Institute of the University of Pennsylvania have proved that glucose causes diabetes, due to its destructive effects on the pancreas. There should be little risk of this if you limit its use to race or game days and for exceptionally long training sessions.

Many endurance athletes consume white sugar by the pound in cola drinks, candy bars, cookies and homemade drinks. What does it do to the body?

Yudkin, to put the worst first, says cancer and leukemia have been statistically correlated with high sugar consumption.

Anthropologists find few cavities in the teeth of skulls uncovered in excavating prehistoric sites. There is little disagreement among researchers that tooth decay is a product of the "modern" sweet—white sugar. Native children in sugar-producing countries chew unrefined raw sugar cane all day and get few cavities.

Sugar has been implicated in acne, though there are other causes for this skin disease of toxin elimination. Gout is another disease suspected to have a causal connection with high sugar consumption.

Deficiencies of the B vitamins, which have serious importance for the athlete, are associated with eating refined sugar, which requires some of these vitamins for its digestion. Since the natural vitamins of the sugar cane or beet are removed in refining, white sugar leaches the body's stores of vitamin B without replacing them.

Notice that we've used "refined" and "white" to refer to the whole class of industrial sugars. But these also include those sugars which are commonly thought to be healthier than the pure-white version: "kleenraw," "brown," "dark brown," etc.

The most disastrous effect of white sugar on the athlete's body is its interference with the delicate mechanisms of energy production. Because of what scientists already know about sugar's interference with the enzyme chains through which food is turned into energy, Yudkin speculates that "over many years, a continuation of a high-sugar diet results in a decreased ability of the cells properly to use their ordinary metabolic materials such as glucose, for which they require hormones, especially insulin."

HEAT

Apologists for the standard American diet will tell you man has lived for thousands of years on cooked food, that his body has therefore adapted itself to using cooked foods as efficiently as a raw diet. A "good hot meal" is supposed to be just the thing for protection from winter cold and to give you brimming energy for training. Yet this idea has no basis in human physiology, since the chemical reactions that convert food into energy do not require the extra heat of cooking. It takes at least a half hour for food to pass beyond the stomach to the intestines, where it begins to be absorbed for energy. By this time its temperature has dropped to that of the surrounding body environment—about 98.6°F. It may feel good to put a warm lump in your stomach on a cold winter day—like an inner hot water bottle—but the heat of cooking does not add one whit to defending you from the cold. Digestion is a chemical process which requires no contribution of heat from outside the body.

Earlier we quoted Dr. Ernst van Aaken's remark that the athlete of the future will be an "enzyme athlete"—that is, conscious of the enormous importance of enzymes in his or her metabolism. Possibly the most destructive effect of heat on food concerns enzymes.

When our body temperature rises above 106-107° we die—because our body's enzymes are damaged at such high temperatures. Our food is similarly "killed" by heat: body temperature causes enzymes to work more rapidly, but above 120°F all the enzymes in food are destroyed. Hygienist C.E. Burtis writes that enzymes "initiate the conversion of raw materials into body cells, store glycogen in the liver and muscles, change carbohydrates into fat, proteins into fats and sugars, aid in the excretion of the by-products of digestion and carry out a host of complex changes without which the life processes would come to a complete halt.

"A curious phenomenon, illustrative of the vital importance of raw foods in the diet, is the appearance of leucocytes in the digestive tract during the digestion of a meal of cooked foods. Since leucocytes (white blood cells) normally appear at the site of an infection, this indicates that the destruction of normally occurring enzymes by heat results in a condition that is inimical and extremely embarrassing to the digestive functions." Eating raw foods

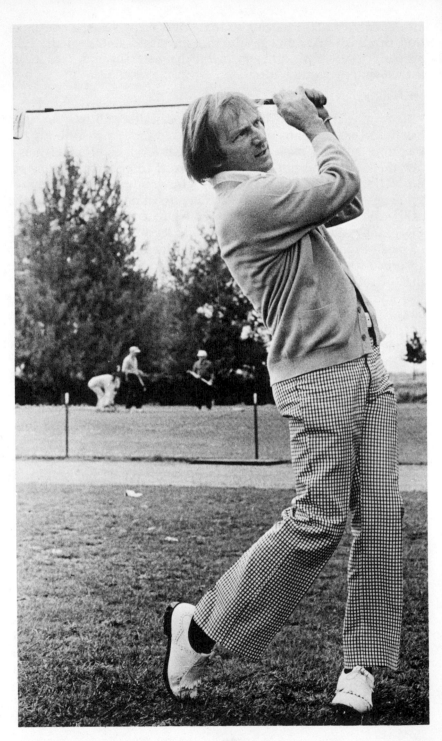

with cooked foods prevents this process to some extent, but if the cooked food has been heated to the temperature of boiling water, adding raw foods won't prevent leucocytosis. '

Proteins are altered to unassimilable forms by heat. This is known to occur during the pasteurization process, during which milk is heated to 140°F for at least an hour, destroying all the enzymes as well. Endocrinologist (gland specialist) Henry Bieler, M.D. says, "Milk is one of the most unstable, thermolabile (damaged by heat) of all the natural foods. Even refrigeration for 24 hours will rob it of some of its vitamin content and its organic structure. Pasteurization disintegrates it still more, while boiling reduces it to a useless, putrefiable mess that is tolerated by the liver with great difficulty . . . Despite the reverence for Pasteur, enlightened pediatricians know that pasteurization of cow's milk for infant feeding is a definitely harmful process. The large dairy interests use pasteurization to ensure preservation, to keep milk from souring quickly . . . But cleanly handled milk need not be pasteurized, as is proved by the excellent quality and sweetness of certified raw milk. When available, it should always be used."

Lysine is one of the most important amino acids in protein foods. It is damaged by heat, and this results in the body being unable to properly utilize other amino acids. The end product of such incomplete metabolism, says C.E. Burtis, "being highly toxic, creates a twin problem of malnutrition and toxemia."

Starchy foods that have been heated have been found to contain a cancer-causing chemical, 3-4 benzophrene. Overheated fats are also suspected of causing cancer. They are found in great numbers of processed foods.

Herbert Shelton, the most brilliant living hygienist, presents a detailed review of the research on heat's effects on food in his book *Orthotrophy, Vol. II.* He lists the main findings:

1. Cooking coagulates (hardens) the proteins of milk, meat, eggs, etc., making them tough and, with the exception of egg protain, less digestible, while impairing their food values.

2. Cooking alters the fats in foods, rendering them less digestible and converting some of them into poisons.

3. Cooking causes a great loss of the soluble minerals in the food.

Fluid electrolytes in hot weather, vitamins and enzymes for vision and mental/muscular coordination, freedom from digestive disturbances—all are factors in shooting low golf scores.

4. Cooking destroys the elementary plant form, tearing down its structure, changing its composition and bringing about certain destructive changes in the element-groupings in all foods, returning part of these elements, especially the organic salts, to their inorganic, and therefore useless, state, so that a large part of their mineral content is lost.

5. Cooking renders starches less digestible and more prone to fermentation.

6. Cooking destroys the vitamins in foods and impairs or completely destroys their anti-neuritic, anti-scorbutic, etc., factors.

7. Cooking drives off part of the food into the air as gases. Eggs and vegetables like cabbage which are rich in sulphur, have their sulphur oxidized. They should never be cooked. Phosphorus is also oxidized. The iron is ruined as food. Iodine and manganese are oxidized at low temperatures.

In a famous experiment, scientist Francis Pottenger fed 900 cats on varied raw and cooked diets for 10 years. Cats receiving raw meat and raw milk remained perfectly healthy and gave birth normally. Cats receiving cooked meats as the major portion of their diet became ill. They had great difficulty in birth and their kittens were sickly and diseased.

C.E. Burtis reports that the females of the Pottenger experiment who'd been fed cooked meat were "vicious and dangerous to handle; the males—and here we may have a clue to the behavior of a considerable segment of the male population in the human species today—were listless, docile, spiritless . . . Finally, while the raw-meat-fed cats exhibited robust good health generation after generation, the cooked-meat-fed cats died out in the third generation of the experiment—*none* of the third generation kittens lived more than six months."

We warned you that nothing would be sacred here, that diet reform is a tough challenge to self-respect and ambition. So, here goes the biggest profanation of the sacred we've undertaken so far: even ice cream isn't holy anymore. Dr. Axel Emil Gibson, quoted by Bieler in *Food is Your Best Medicine*, describes what happens to pasteurized milk after it's subjected to the "second insult" of freezing: "The freezing process, however, gives to the cream its last and finishing touch of physiological corruption. Quickly fermenting substances like milk, cream, fruit, etc., break down structurally at the first touch of frost. And, as the arrest of bacterial activities caused by the frost is only temporary while the molecular derangement of the frozen substance remains a permanent menace, it follows that a renewal and increase of the destructive work of the invading microbes immediately takes place when the ice cream reaches its melting point in the stomach . . . so the ice cream, melting in the body of the individual, sets free the carcasses of the ice cream and milk cells, to lay them open to the resistless attacks of swarming and festering bacteria—though the evidence of the ghostly carnival of putrefaction escapes the taste by being masked into unrecognizability by the great deceiver—sugar."

Recent studies have found the Salk polio vaccine to be far less effective than it was initially thought, if not completely worthless. In support of the idea that polio may be linked to diet, Dr. Bieler cites a study conducted in Asheville, North Carolina by a Dr. Benjamin F. Sandler. "During one summer, the children ate no sweets whatsoever. In previous years, a large number of polio cases had occurred during the summer season. But, during the summer of Dr. Sandler's experiment, significantly enough, there were 90 percent fewer cases. Naturally, avoiding all sweets included avoiding ice cream. But if other kinds of sweet food were as dangerous, surely epidemics of polio would follow Christmas and Easter. As we know, this is not what happens. Inevitably, the finger of suspicion points strongly toward the villain—ice cream."

Bieler recommends that parents substitute fresh cold homemade desserts for ice cream, for example a mixture of fresh whipped cream, honey and crushed fruit. He warns that it shouldn't be eaten with meals as the combination is overtaxing to the liver, and that it should be chilled in the refrigerator rather than frozen.

We're not talking about performance-specific nutrition here, so it may seem like we've strayed from the subject of food for fitness. But whether subtle in the form of metabolic inefficiency, or acute in illnesses that really lay us low, there is no doubt that disease hampers performance. And the reward of diet-assisted positive health is far greater than mere absence of disease. The people who compiled this book have followed its suggestions, and can testify from firsthand personal experience that health is positive attainment—something *added* in vitality, alertness and energy, and not just a status quo carefully defended against the advance of disease.

WHITE FLOUR

James Turner points out in *The Chemical Feast* that food industry executives like white flour better than rats and insects do. Pests avoid it as insufficiently nutritious to support life. White flour keeps on the shelf longer than its whole wheat relative, but the price for long shelf life is the stripping of 22 nutrients from the "staff of life." Only four of these are reinstated during the so-called enrichment process, but the food value of white flour remains almost nil, since the "enrichment" vitamins are usually unassimilable inorganic chemicals in unbalanced amounts and combinations.

The *Newsletter* of the Academy of Applied Nutrition noted the ironical fact that since white flour keeps longer, whole wheat bread may actually be even less nutritious by the time it reaches the consumer: "Test animals, consequently, survived better on white bread than they did on commercial whole wheat bread. There were *no* survivors among the animals fed on commercial whole wheat bread." The solution? Most health food stores keep their bread under refrigeration from the moment it's delivered by the bakery. Or, you can make your own inexpensive, delicious whole wheat bread with fresh-milled flour. If you're really serious about health you might try Christ's recipe for "sun-cooked" wheat bread, in *The Essene Gospel of Peace:*

> Moisten your wheat, that the angel of water may enter it. Then set it in the air, that the angel of air also may embrace it. And leave it from morning to evening beneath the sun, that the angel of sunshine may descend upon it. And the blessing of the three angels will soon make the germ of life to sprout in your wheat. Then crush your grain, and make thin wafers, as did your forefathers when they departed out of Egypt, the house of bondage. Put them back again beneath the sun from its appearing, and when it is risen to its highest in the heavens, turn them over on the other side that they be embraced there also by the angel of sunshine, and leave them there until the sun be set. For the angels of water, of air, and of sunshine fed and ripened the wheat in the field, and they, likewise, must prepare also your bread. (*The Essene Gospel of Peace*, Academy Books, 3085 Reynard Way, San Diego, Calif.)

And finally, white flour acts like glue in the intestines, severely inhibiting the absorption of food through the intestinal lining. A Massachusetts coroner found in over 200 autopsies only two or three truly healthy intestinal tracts. The vast majority were so compacted with indescribable filth that there was only a tiny, finger-sized passage through which food could travel—hardly the best conditions for efficient absorption of nutrients, and traced by the coroner in question chiefly to the "gumming" qualities of

The body at its concentrated best. You may not need to carbohydrate load for short events like the hurdles, but diet errors will take their toll on the "fine tuning" with which you go to the starting line. (John Marconi Photo)

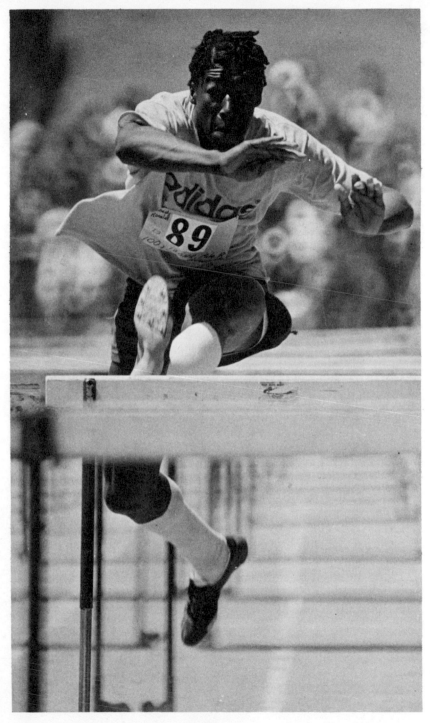

white flour. Many of the tracts contained worms of up to 2½ feet in length, which could not have lived in the clean environment created by efficient digestion and lack of putrefaction from wrong eating.

How about boxed breakfast cereals? *Consumer Bulletin,* November 1961, found packaged cereals overpriced, with dangerous amounts of the amino acid lysine added in some cases, or of negligible value as food due to the high temperatures used in processing. Added sugar makes them worse, and they are subject to all the pollution problems of any grain: "Sour, decomposed, insect-infested grains and grains polluted by rodent excreta are common," reported *CB*. "Cyanides are extensively used in the treatment of cereal crops of all kinds for control of insect infestations, and a sizeable residue of cyanide and of various bromides is permitted in the finished grain."

C.E. Burtis recommends, ". . . best of all, if your chewing mechanism is not impaired, after soaking and liquefying, eat them [whole grains] as is with cream and fruit."

INORGANIC SUBSTANCES

Salt is the first to come to mind. "How can salt be a food when it passes through the body unchanged," asks hygienist Shelton, "being ejected from all of the ejector organs in the same state in which it is taken into the stomach? If it is taken into the stomach as salt, hurried through the system as salt and cast out as salt, how in the name of bread-and-butter can it nourish the tissues?" Shelton reminds us that the North American indians did not employ salt until taught to do so by the white man. Rommel's troops in North Africa during World War II survived the desert heat very well without salt.

The Holyoke marathon of 1968 was a terrible ordeal. This national championship event at the 26-mile, 385-yard Olympic marathon distance was started—quite stupidly—at noon in over-90° heat. The favorites dropped out like flies. Two national class runners who survived in good condition discovered after the race that they had one thing in common: both of them had eliminated salt from their diet, and had since noticed that they ran very well in hot weather.

Workers in the hot fields of Arizona and Israel were tested in a study by Schamadan and Snively. This study and another conducted by Kenneth Cooper of the famous Aerobics Institute, concurred that the main electrolytes lost in hot weather physical work are potassium and magnesium, not sodium.

Two very important points should be mentioned concerning salt. When an athlete actually nears heat prostration his body suddenly starts dumping sodium at a phenomenal rate. In heat collapse the very *best* treatment is a 3% salt water solution. This has been used by marathon trainer van Aaken for years with total success. Dr. van Aaken cites terrifying cases of distance runners being given pure water by ignorant medical personnel and dying from the resulting further dilution of their body's electrolytes.

The other important point concerns the fact that an athlete will never drink enough to "bring his body fluid level up to par" following a hot race or game. It will normally take several days before the athlete, following his or her natural desire to drink, replaces fluid losses. Some physiologists mistakenly advise forcing ourselves to drink more than we desire. This is nonsense, as it is obvious that the body must first be allowed to replace its lost electrolytes through eating before it can be given more liquid, so that the already depleted supply isn't diluted still further.

Henry Bieler, M.D. had studied the evils of salt for over 30 years at the time of writing *Food is Your Best Medicine*. He lists three stages of "salt poisoning" in the person who showers his food with sodium chloride: ". . . in the first, the liver or kidneys or skin, or all three, may show functional derangement, followed (second stage) by organic destruction. Albumen, casts, red blood cells and pus in the urine—all signs of extensive kidney destruction—may usher in the third stage of salt poisoning." Bieler asks, "Why not, then, let the plants synthesize NaCl into an organic form, in their leaves and fruits and roots and stems, and eat it that way? A simple solution, isn't it? The urine and sweat never show an excess of salt when it is consumed in this form."

Many useless inorganic substances in the modern diet are ballyhooed as "enrichments" by food manufacturers. "Drug store iron, for example, is of no value in anemia," says Herbert Shelton. "If there is any deficiency of any nutrient in our body, this must be supplied in the proper form or it will not be assimilated in tissue building . . . It is possible to analyze an apple and ascertain its chemical constituents; but all the chemists in the world cannot make an apple, nor anything that can substitute for it. There must be a vegetable arrangement of these elements, else they are wholly innutritious. Only the plant can take the raw materials of soil, water and air, and with the use of the sun, synthesize suitable substances for animal nutrition." The "jiffy meal in a convenient food stick" is a dangerous delusion of the food industry.

Several years ago fluoridation of water for the purpose of preventing tooth decay became the center of a great controversy.

Scientific studies gave evidence of its harmlessness, while right radicals called it a communist plot. Leonard Wickendan has now summarized the arguments against fluorides in his book *Our Daily Poison.* He cites recent evidence of fluorides' damaging cumulative effects on kidneys, liver and heart.

All the chemical additives are, of course, unphysiologic materials, and less than half of the 2500 currently in use have been tested for safety. Evidence is growing in support of the general principle that what doesn't do the body any nutritional good, should be left alone.

CANCER

Hygienists have maintained for years that cancer is nutrition-related, and some evidence from research laboratories is now pointing strongly in the same direction. Max Gerson, a researcher and physician who operated a cancer clinic, wrote in *A Cancer Therapy* (Whittier Books): "Cancer is not a local but a general disease, caused chiefly by the poisoning of foodstuffs prepared by modern farming and food industry." Gerson is supported by the fact that 75 years ago cancer was a rare disease.

Studies of cancer-free populations reveal that though their diets vary, all live on simple foods—"of good quality, adequate in quantity; and they were *whole* diets. That is, their foods were natural, unsophisticated, untouched or unchanged by processing or refinement, and of high biological quality." (Burtis)

The Nader FDA study points out that many of the food additives whitewashed by the Food and Drug Administration are suspected cancer-producing substances. Burtis also discusses the connection at length, and his book is recommended reading on the topic of diet and cancer.

Dr. Bieler refers to "a dictionary-sized book on cancer and diet" (title unfortunately not known to us) written by Dr. Frederick Hoffman, for many years chief statistician for Prudential Life Insurance Co., who concluded: "I am fully convinced that profound dietary influences in cancer are to be looked upon as a causative factor."

The literature of hygiene is full of cases of cancer cures following upon fasting under experienced guidance, and radical diet reform. Dr. Bieler was successful in treating many cases by having the patient detoxify his body on a strict drugless high-quality diet, the mainstay of which is "Bieler broth," "a combination of lightly cooked string beans, celery, zucchini and parsley or whatever other vegetables I've recommended for their particular ailments."

INNER POLLUTION

In *Food Combining Made Easy*, Herbert Shelton talks about the dangerous effects of poor assimilation of foods which, left to rot in the intestines, release poisons into the rest of the system:

> When starches and complex sugars are digested they are broken down into simple sugars called monosaccharides, which are usable substances—*nutrients*. When starches and sugars undergo fermentation they are broken down into carbon dioxide, acetic acid, alcohol and water, which substances, with the exception of water, are non-usable substances—*poisons*. When proteins are digested, they are broken down into amino acids, which are usable substances—*nutrients*. When proteins putrefy, they are broken down into a variety of ptomaines and leucomaines, which are non-usable substances—*poisons*. So with all other food factors—enzymic digestion of foods prepares them for use by the body. The first process gives us nutrient elements as the finished product; the the second process gives us poisons as the end-result.
>
> What avails it to consume the theoretically required number of calories daily, only to have the food ferment and putrefy in the digestive tract? Food that thus spoils does not yield up its calories to the body. What is gained by eating abundantly of adequate proteins only to have these putrefy in the gastro-intestinal canal? Proteins thus rendered unfit for entrance into the body do not yield up their amino acids. What benefit does one receive from eating vitamin-rich foods only to have these decompose in the stomach and intestines?

As Shelton says, "The causes of digestive inefficiency and failure are legion." They include fatigue, hot weather, drinking alcohol, bad food combinations and worry—to name only a tiny handful. Here again we'll have to admit we just don't have space to cover the topic adequately. The principles of digestive efficiency are quite simple and easy to learn, even though the opportunities for error sound distressingly complex.

The single most common cause of intestinal putrefaction is poor food combining. World Publications carries Shelton's *Food Combining Made Easy*, and it's one of Shelton's works which we recommend unreservedly. We've tried food combining ourselves and have found it really makes a difference in vitality, athletic performance, and the complete absence of "after-meal slump."

We're down to the end of this catch-all discussion of food dangers and errors. Once again, please don't be "freaked" by the seeming complexity of it all. Complex problems only arise when nature is ignored. Her rules are strict and unyielding, but simple.

Food habits need not be changed overnight. To return to simplicity takes time. First give yourself a chance to *learn*, if you are dissatisfied with your status quo and desire to change. Knowledge is your best weapon against old habits and temptation. If you're firmly convinced that a thing will harm you there's nothing in the world that will make you eat it.

Take the long view. Say you've spent 20 years eating junk foods. If you take 10 years to improve your diet—even just changing one small item every six months—most likely the remainder of your life will be longer and more pleasant for your gradual efforts. Some people dive right into diet reform and make radical changes without batting an eyelash, but for many of us the slower way works best.

The chapter of this book on changing habits was written out of the realization that dietary revolution is as difficult as it is indispensable for best health and performance. Don't throw up your hands in despair—diet reform really *is* possible, and immensely rewarding. You have a *right* to enjoy the maximum vitality and pure unhindered efficiency of which your body is capable. Seize that right and no longer be the victim of old, past misconceptions and societal pressures. Just remember the prod to pride given by James Rorty and N. Phillip Norman, M.D. in their book *Bio-Organics:* "Bad food habits are not immaculately conceived as a kind of Original .Anthropological Sin. They are a form of conditioned individual and group social behavior, as a result of which a lot of very poor people get beri-beri and pellagra and a few quite rich people make a lot of money."

THE FACTS ABOUT PROTEIN

by Dr. Ralph Bircher

Dr. Ralph Bircher is director of the world-famous Bircher-Benner Clinic in Zurich, Switzerland.

> *Believe those who seek the truth;*
> *suspect those who have found it.*
> —André Gide

Gide's admonition seems to me nowhere more applicable than in the controversy over protein. In the research literature which it has been my duty to examine critically and impartially for the last 40 years, I have seen the most respectable kind of work mixed with a shameful pile of ignorance—much of it by "respected" au-

thors—such as I've encountered in no other scientific
conclusions contradict so fantastically that one finds hi
ing his head in despair. Medical textbooks naturally d
the uncertainty of the situation: textbooks merely r
monly-held prejudices, and a lot doesn't appear in th
simple reason that "what *may* not be, *must* not be!"

HOW MUCH?

First the basic question: "How much protein does a human
being need to stay healthy and perform well? What are the daily
requirements, the minimum, the optimum, for a standard body
weight of 154 pounds?"

The respected authorities at the turn of the century were
Rubner and Voit, who said we needed 120–160 grams per day.
Chittenden then showed in human experiments that best performance and health were assured on 50 grams.   Hinhede set the
figure at 30.

Today, after a quarter of a century during which mountains
of protein research papers have been published, the situation is no
better. In Russia, Jakovlev set up a minimum requirement of 144–
163 grams.   Kuhnau put the optimum at 200.   Kofranyi of the
Max Planck Institute proved that complete nitrogen balance and
performance capacity could be maintained on 25 grams, and
Oomen and Hipsley found a population that develop robust health
on a mere 15–20 grams with magnificent muscular structure and excellent physical performance. Elvehjem insists that the optimum
amount is quite near the minimum—that is, no great "margin of
safety" is advisable.

The American Research Council's Food and Nutrition Board
agreed on a daily requirement for adults of 70 grams—the number
currently found in most tables. Sherman, a member of the Board,
told how this figure was arrived at. The evidence had pointed to a
much lower figure, around 35 grams. But Board members feared
that if the requirement were set so low there would be a public
outcry—and certainly protests from the meat and dairy industries.
And so, a corresponding "margin of safety" was adopted. Since
scientific backing was absent for the 70-gram figure the word "re-
commendation" was used, instead of "requirement."

In practice, everybody thought 70 grams was the *minimum*—
in spite of research indicating that excessive protein intake is harmful to health.

ONE MAN'S MEAT—ANOTHER MAN'S WHEAT

No less confusing is the matter of protein quality, and

...ier animal or plant protein is preferable. The textbooks say
...getable protein is inferior—at least a third of the protein intake
...supposedly must come from animal sources. (The public auto-
matically thinks "meat" when they read "animal sources," though
there *are* such things as milk and eggs!)

The presumed inferiority of vegetable protein lacks scientific
proof. If scientists had studied the geography and history of nutrition with the thoroughness they applied to their chemical and
animal experiments, they would never have fallen into this dogma.
There are now populations numbering in the millions in various
parts of the earth of whom it is known from penetrating research
that they have developed enviable health and strength for thousands of years on a purely vegetarian diet. McCollum, discoverer
of vitamin D, showed in 1923 the high protein quality of a whole
wheat and green vegetable combination. Abelin reported the same
results in 1942 in the Swiss medical journal. According to Verzar
in 1956, 10 different purely vegetable protein combinations of the
highest biological quality were known to the Food and Agriculture
Organization of the UN.

Only in the last few years was it demonstrated at the Max
Planck Institute for Nutritional Physiology that the previous bases
for calculation, which had shown animal protein to be essential,
were erroneous.

Under the old practice, the protein under investigation was
considered only as useful as the amino acid which was least strongly represented in it. In reality, though, proteins are hardly ever
eaten one at a time, but always combined, thus reinforcing one
another. The old method was "not just unproved, but simply in-
valid." (Kofra, NYI). Biological quality is always significantly
higher in combinations—thus the non-essential amino acids have a
decisive importance not previously suspected or explained.

The protein of corn and beans, combined in a ratio of 55:
45%, is equal in quality to the best egg protein. The protein combination of 500 grams of potatoes with 50 grams of chicken egg
is considerably higher in biological quality than egg, milk or meat
protein alone. Health can be maintained on less than 25 grams of
protein a day using this combination.

To date only combinations of two protein sources have been
tested. We can't discount the possibility that combinations of
three or more sources will show even higher values.

There is a further possibility that the body benefits from bacterial proteins in the nitrogen in the air. This is the only possible
explanation for the findings of Oomen and Hipsley among the
equatorial highlanders of New Guinea, who get an average of 15—

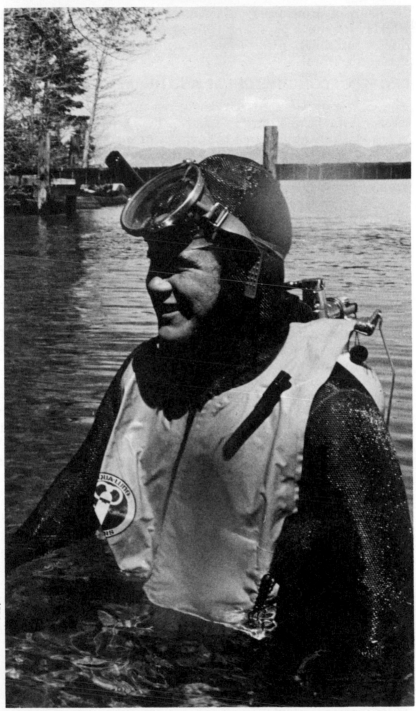

20 grams of protein per day and yet are exceptionally healthy, work at strenuous physical labor and develop athletic body structures. Just think of the vistas opened up for world nutrition by these discoveries!

PROTEIN ECONOMY: CHEAP AND HEALTHY

Obviously we need not reduce our protein intake to similar levels. If we bring it down to half of the current excess—say, 50 grams—we can rest assured of a sufficient margin of safety. The first law of nutritional economy is that every excess of food and calories—particularly excess protein—works not to a person's advantage but to the deterioration of his health.

Protein deficiency is the major malnutrition problem worldwide, but it is not the only problem. If we moderate our concepts of protein's importance to 50 grams and concentrate on total nutritional needs, our nutritional foreign aid will be more effective. We'll stop feeding starving children protein concentrates that are completely useless as long as the child's *total* diet isn't correspondingly normalized. We'll stop sending milk powder to Africa to be used as whitewash after it produces severe indigestion.

Another consequence of eating only 50 grams a day will be that we'll no longer need *any* protein-rich foods. Potatoes, for example, contain barely 2% protein, but of the highest quality—equal to that of eggs. In combination with small amounts of egg protein, potato protein is of the very highest value. Potato protein alone is sufficient for long periods of time, in spite of its low content in percentage figures. Test subjects eating potato as their sole source of protein remained healthy and strong for five and a half months. The addition of some animal protein does, of course, constitute a guarantee.

THE RAW FACTS

People make mistakes when they become fanatical and do not know the facts. The quality of and requirement for protein depend on several factors; for instance, on heating, which can considerably lower the quality of protein. The usual heating of meats results in a significant decrease in essential amino acids. The same is true of drying and conserving, as in the pasteurization of milk. It probably isn't socially acceptable to eat raw meat, but eating other raw foods contributes greatly to reducing the total volume of protein that must be eaten.

Raw food decreases the need for protein in still another way. The standard diet requires 6–8 grams of protein per day just for the synthesis of digestive juices. But raw food digests itself, thanks to its enzyme content.

Protein economy begins with the feeding of babies. In the early '50's nature failed the test of American medicine. It was found that breast milk "contains 60% less protein than the infant needs." A "formula" was created with two and a half to three times the protein, plus added salt. Today we know it wasn't nature but an incautious science that failed. Mother Nature was avenged by devastating consequences: kidney damage, hyperacidity with osteoporosis, dangerously high phenylalanine and tyrosine levels in the blood, poor protein metabolism, and accelerated growth which produced a stressful inharmony between physical and mental development.

"PROTEIN POWER" FOR ATHLETES?

A physiological poison which has been isolated and traced to meat eating is uric acid, a very strong irritant on the sympathetic nerves. Stimulation has traditionally contributed to meat's reputation as "strength food"—far in excess of its actual nutritive value. Continuous excitation of the nerves, which seems to be considered a necessity of life in these times, is no sign of *strength*. It stands in the way of the regenerative work of the nervous system. This is the main reason why in hygienic therapy we renounce all stimulants including meat.

Regeneration and recovery demand detoxification and metabolic economy. This is particularly true in athletics, where the last degree of performance must be extracted. The advantages of a meatless diet show up with special clarity in high mountain work, as a 10–20% reduction in oxygen requirement and a 30% lower caloric requirement with correspondingly improved performance, recovery and adaptive capacity.

Indian populations living at 13,000 feet in the Andes highlands hold stubbornly to an ancient protein economy in spite of well-meant advice from the World Health Organization. They race bicycles for distances of 150 miles at average speeds of 25 mph. Similarly, the Tarahumara indians of Mexico run 90 miles at seven mph with no heart expansion or shortness of breath. Experience has taught these highland people to stick to protein economy.

Even rats that were taken to high altitudes suffered deficiencies in nutritional utilization on a high-protein diet, but not on low protein fare. The detrimental effects of an excess-protein diet occur at sea level also, but they have immediate practical significance in the high mountains.

PROTEIN FOR A YOUNG, SLEEK BODY?

The protein question took a new turn with the recent rise of amyloidose research. Schwarz, a professor of physiological pathology at Frankfurt, described amyloid, a waxy protein mixture, as "the most important and perhaps decisive cause of health decline with age."

It is clear that amyloid consists exclusively of degenerate protein reduction by-products—most likely the result of eating excess protein which must be quickly burned but cannot be sufficiently eliminated.

All the essential amino acids, especially the sulphurous ones, can cause damage when eaten to excess. Even on just 70 grams of protein a day containing all the essential amino acids there can be a harmful intake of some of the amino acids. The connection between amyloidosis and excess protein is easily proved by animal experiment. Amyloid contains rich amounts of the amino acids tryptophane and tyrosine. Five to 10 times as much tryptophane and five to seven times as much tyrosine are found in the dry substances of meat as in vegetable protein sources.

Investigations at Harvard showed that excessive amounts of the amino acid methionine favored hardening of the arteries. Excesses of tryptophane—as mentioned, seven to 10 times as richly present in meat and eggs as in plants—are eagerly consumed by cancer cells which make serotonin from it, producing severe disturbances in the organism. (Smoking also blocks tryptophane metabolism, leading to a great increase in cancer-producing ortho-aminophenols.)

PROTEIN AND THE MINERAL BANK

Bone decay (bone atrophy or osteoporosis) is extraordinarily widespread in modern man. It begins in childhood and is spreading rapidly. Extensive scientific literature deals with its possible causes. Wachmann and Bernstein of Harvard reported the results of all previous research in the prestigious medical journal *Lancet* and concluded that protein-rich—in particular, meat-heavy—diet plays the strongest role in causing osteoporosis.

Bone atrophy is caused when the function of the bone system as a reservoir of basic minerals is continually overstrained. This coincides with the fact that athletes who eat much meat are especially susceptible to arthrosis. Heiss found among 20 professional soccer players who were observed for 18 years 100% incidence of ankle arthrosis and 97.5% incidence of knee arthrosis.

A negative calcium balance is easily produced in experimental animals by increased protein supply, and the animals die of calcium deficiency-associated diseases. The Walker group found among Bantu tribesmen almost no signs of calcium deficiency or weakening of the bones on an almost purely plant-source, protein-poor diet.

The eminent importance of potassium and magnesium is emphasized by several authors. These two basic minerals are deficient in an everyday diet rich in meat, eggs, cheese, fat, sugar and grains, but are abundant in a full-value diet rich in vegetables and raw foods. Potassium and magnesium have been isolated as the most important minerals lost during athletic competition, especially in hot weather.

Animal protein-rich diet and alcohol consumption both hinder the absorption of magnesium from the intestine and correspondingly raise the magnesium requirement. The "magnesium deficiency syndrome" includes arteriosclerosis, high blood pressure, migraine, eclampsia, leaching of calcium from teeth and bones, liver damage and disturbances of the neuromuscular vessel system (Holtmeyer).

Since the early '50's when protein- and salt-enriched artificial baby foods were introduced, athletic medical services in the US have had to treat an extraordinary number of kidney injuries and kidney breakdowns after athletic competition. The American Heart Association concluded that "almost all instances of these diseases [arteriosclerosis, high blood pressure and coronary disease] are significantly related to the kidneys," and that therefore, "more than half of the population die of kidney disease."

VEGGIES AND B$_{12}$

These few aspects of the protein question—we could easily go on—all seem to call for greater attention and further research. Let us briefly mention vitamin B$_{12}$. A greater availability of B$_{12}$ is always cited as evidence of the need for eating meat. But the American Meat Institute's own research, conducted by biochemist Schweigert, showed that the need for B$_{12}$ rises and falls with the amount of protein eaten. Thus, in a protein-economical diet it is correspondingly low. Schweigert also found that whole grain is a usable source of B$_{12}$—if it is not processed into white flour. It would otherwise not have been possible for the hundreds of millions of people who've lived on almost exclusively vegetarian diets to survive without breaking down from B$_{12}$ deficiency.

PROTEIN ECOLOGY

The individual has almost no effect on changing the pollution situation. But he can put the defense and detoxification organs of his own body in the best possible conditon first by detoxify-

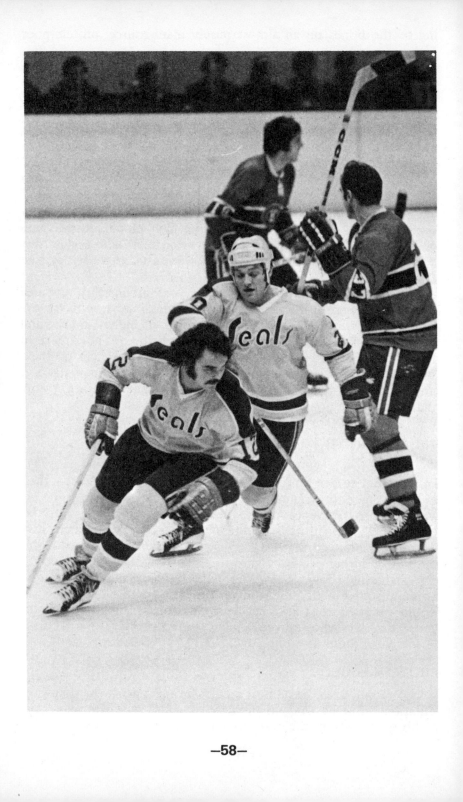

ing the body with fasting and occasional juice diets, and then by making it more powerfully reactive by dietary economy and raw food. We *must* consider that meat and eggs have been far more contaminated since the 1950's than milk and plant products, as a result of conversion to industrial food production methods. Anyone who fully understands the extent to which meat, for example, is treated will certainly think seriously about foregoing it and its by-products. Meat, under the approving eye of the FDA, is currently treated with: tetracyclin, choramphenicol, estrogen, tranquilizers, arsenicals, thyreostatica, tenderizers, conservatives, plus metabolic toxins of the fattening process.

What Serham wrote 20 years ago applies now with far greater intensity: "Feeding grain and potatoes to animals represents an enormous waste of nutritional production potential; and more than that, every person with a social and international sense of justice must become most deeply conscious of the fact that our excessive meat and egg consumption is a leftover from times of colonial exploitation habits . . . If we ourselves do not see the provocative injustice in this situation for poorer classes and peoples, *they* are certainly going to be feeling it with increased intensity. "

Alertness, protection from the cold, fuel for long, hard action and uninterrupted mental stresses make carbohydrate—rich diet and an optimal supply of vitamins, minerals and trace elements essential for the professional ice hockey player. (OMPhoto)

3

The Weight Question

by Dr. Creig Hoyt

Sumo wrestlers gorge themselves on diets exceeding 10,000 calories per day, apparently oblivious to the inevitable price of this orgy—diabetes, hypertension and a life expectancy 10 years less than other Japanese men. An already trim collegiate wrestler fasts for two days and climaxes his drive to "make weight" by sitting in a steam room for 30 minutes before weigh-in. A marathoner keeps his calorie consumption to less than 2500 calories per day to maintain his ultra-lean fitness.

Weight plays a central role in the conditioning of many athletes. It is true that Minnesota Fats was a great billiards star despite his grotesque girth, and Jack Nicklaus a superb golfer even in his fat, sloppy days. Yet, for most athletic activities, weight gain or loss is often a serious concern for participating athletes. Some of the rapid methods of losing weight are perhaps as detrimental to one's health as the perverse obesity of Sumo giants and some professional footballers.

It is naive to think that athletes will forgo these radical alterations in body weight just because physicians counsel against it. Thus, though in this article we will consider both weight loss and gain, and their effect on athletic performance, I must emphasize that the discussion of these practices is not an endorsement by me; my own opinion is that the vast majority of Americans are overweight, and their health suffers from it. Furthermore, most crash diets do not produce long-lasting weight reduction, and are not beneficial to one's overall health. Be that as it may, let us consider the benefits of weight alterations in various activities.

REGULATION OF FOOD INTAKE

The precise nature of what signals the body that it is, or should be, "hungry" is not yet known. It is established that there are several different signals that the body may respond to in perceiving whether it should take in more or less food. The central monitoring area of all these signals is probably the hypothalamus— a region of the brain where many complex body functions are processed. From animal studies we know that the lateral portion of the hypothalamus is a feeding center responsible for the urge to eat; the medial portion of the hypothalamus has a contrasting area which exerts an inhibitory control over the feeding center— this is a "satiety" center. The types of input to the hypothalamus are varied and not fully understood. However, the following aspects are discussed in order to give the reader an idea of the complexity of the biological events which go towards constituting "hunger" or "satiety."

Several studies have emphasized that a central role is played by the blood sugar level in regulating food intake. There is, no doubt, a strong protective mechanism to maintain adequate glucose at the cellular level. Thus, the hypothalamus responds to hypoglycemia (low blood sugar) with a signal of intense hunger. However, whether it is the actual blood sugar level or some secondary hormonal change which signals the brain is not clear. The blood sugar effect on appetite is probably an extraordinarily complex interaction of several hormonal and neural systems.

Another prominent interaction of the food intake system is that which takes place with heat exchange. An elevation of body temperature inhibits the sensation of hunger, a fact most of us have experienced during periods of intense physical activity. The opposite effect is also well known to most of us—when body temperature falls, the hunger sensation becomes manifest. Many of us fight the weight battle during winter as a result.

It has been suggested by some researchers that the nutritive value of ingested foods is evaluated by gastric sensors which relay the information to the hypothalamus. This has been invoked as the ultimate explanation for the suppression of appetite that occurs with ingestion of fats. How extensive this "evaluation" system is has yet to be determined. Nevertheless, I think you can see that the reactions which control "hunger" are extremely complex in nature. In addition, many studies have emphasized that these factors express themselves quite differently in different age groups, cultural groups, and between the sexes.

"IDEAL" WEIGHT

The notion of an "ideal" weight is an intellectual construct without any real point of reference. One of the better known norms is the one first published by the Metropolitan Life Insurance Company. In actual fact it is nothing more than an averaging of a large group of Americans examined upon application for insurance policies. This type of "ideal" weight table is obviously an average of what people weigh, not necessarily what they should "ideally" weigh.

There is very little basic research data to firmly establish an "ideal" weight in terms of one that would be most healthful. The need for a simple but meaningful method of assessing body composition, including the amount of adipose tissue (fat), is apparent. Several methods have been used including anthropometric measurement, skin-fold thickness, body densitometry, total body potassium levels, and radial-ulnar diameter measurements. I think that specific gravity measurements are most meaningful to the majority of athletes.

In one study of 25 professional footballers, 17 were deemed overweight according to standard height-weight tables. Yet, 11 of the 17 had excessively high lean body masses as measured by specific gravity determinations. Thus, in sports where muscular over-development is a significant factor in the training process the body weight of the participating athletes may seem quite high though the protein/fat ratio determinations may be quite acceptable. With this type of discussion as a background, it should be obvious that the term "weight" is not what we are really concerned with, but rather it is "body composition." Nonetheless, I shall use the term "weight" throughout the remainder of this article because so much of the data available is really based on "weight." Furthermore, most American amateur athletes do not have access to a center where the more precise types of body composition determinations can be made. Most of us at present are forced to examine our weight in order to make an indirect inference about our actual body composition.

WEIGHT AS AN ENEMY

The great distance runners of the last few decades have been the pioneers in showing the way to other endurance athletes—"get rid of the extra baggage." In sports where prolonged aerobic exercise takes place, the current champions are at incredibly lean body weights. Road cyclists, runners, cross-country skiers, walkers and many others have adopted the lean look. The data on the relationship between aerobic efficiency and body weight are very impressive. In marathon runners it has been shown that maximal aerobic speed increased 5% for each 5% drop in body weight. This type of benefit to aerobic fitness with weight loss is now an established tenet among work physiologists. Thus, there is a large group of athletes conscious of staying trim and/or losing weight to improve aerobic fitness.

Another group of athletes pursues weight reduction for a much less physiologic reason. Many wrestlers and boxers depend on dropping four to five pounds in the final days before competition. As a collegiate wrestler I participated in this unhealthy practice. The reason this is often done is in order that an athlete can compete at a lower weight level than his normal weight—on the thesis that his strength will allow him to dominate his smaller opponents. This is usually nullified by the fact that both competitors are doing the same thing. They starve and sweat the last few days before they meet in battle. Even more absurd is the practice of allowing some "weigh-ins" the night before competition. A 163-pound man can easily lose six pounds of water in the steam room, "make weight" at 157, and be right back at 163 the day of the meet; so, the 157-pound class has two competitors at 163. However, as I said in the preface to this article, my condemnation of this practice will not alter it; so I shall discuss weight loss for this group of athletes as well as for the "endurance" athletes.

For the athlete trying to lose weight in order to improve his aerobic fitness, the best weight reduction program is a gradual one of moderate calorie restriction. Some experiments have shown that if you lose weight at a rate of greater than one-third pound per day, your muscular strength will decline due to this too-rapid loss. Now it is true that with almost any serious reducing diet you will lose four to five pounds in the first two or three days. However, this is not fat but rather water.

Any reducing diet inevitably results in some carbohydrate restriction. Thus, during the initial days of the diet liver glycogen stores are mobilized for energy (the body preferentially utilizes carbohydrates rather than fats for most kinds of activity). Since each gram of glycogen is stored with almost three grams of water, the initial weight loss during this "mobilization" can be impressive. However, these are the pounds which will reappear as you return to a normal diet. So once this initial water loss has taken place, I'd aim for a quarter or a third of a pound of weight reduction daily.

There are many diets advertised as "the way" to trim down. Their great number speaks for their lack of any "magic"; the easy way to lose weight has not been found. Several of the current popular diets (Pennington, Atkins', and Water diet) are based upon severe carbohydrate restriction. This is turn leads to acidosis (lowering of the blood pH) which depresses the appetite center. However, these diets are not acceptable for even moderately active individuals. The depletion of liver glycogen in these diets is so complete that it is extremely difficult to generate glucose for muscular activity. Furthermore, the ketosis (breakdown of fatty acids) and resulting acidosis cause pronounced limitations for attempts at prolonged exercise.

For the serious aerobic-minded athlete calorie restriction can be a much more physiologically sound alternative. Every pound of excess weight represents 4000 calories—calories you must burn up and not replace. Combining calorie restriction with increased activity is my way to lose weight. For example, if you are a 170-pound man and you want to lose 10 pounds, cut your calories and run a bit more. You probably need around 3000 calories to maintian your current weight, so cut it to 2000 calories (not a starvation amount by any means). If you run five miles a day (at any speed), that is another 500 calories per day lost. The total 1500 calories in deficit will put you right on the goal of one-third pound per day loss.

For those athletes who are going to drop several pounds over a short period in order to compete, the method of weight loss must be either salt restriction and external heat, or abstinence from carbohydrates. Either one will promote the rapid water loss required in this crash program. Since most of the athletes who adhere to this tactic are boxers or wrestlers, the essential feature is to drop the weight with as little loss of muscular strength as possible. There is considerable evidence to suggest that salt restriction and heat is preferable to carbohydrate fasting. In severe glycogen-store deficiency it may require up to 24 hours to achieve normal liver stores again; so even if the "weigh-in" is 12 hours prior to competition, the sugar available to muscles will not be normal during the match. On the other hand, dehydration by salt restriction has an effect on endurance, but very little on short anaerobic periods of exercise. Let me emphasize again—I do not endorse either of these methods of sudden weight loss; a weight loss of greater than 2% of your body weight in this acute dehydrating fashion can lead to kidney, muscle, or heart damage.

WEIGHT AS AN ALLY

I have already voiced my opinion that an increase in body weight is rarely a beneficial attribute (in terms of your health), but then again I am not being paid those grossly inflated salaries to bash opposing lines each Sunday. There is no getting around the fact that big-time football now requires most men to be 200 pounds plus. Many field competitors and weight-lifters also desire high body weights. Of course, these athletes do not want excessive fat but hope to develop increased muscle mass (and strength) as the result of their increased weight.

To achieve increased weight (and strength) many different paths have been outlined—high protein diets, androgens, and increased calorie consumption. During the '50's several famous musclemen made protein supplements the fashion. Several thorough studies have shown since then that there is no need to increase protein intake in order to achieve increased muscle mass. Excessive dietary protein is simply broken down into sugar fragments and nitrogen. Thus, in an atmosphere of soaring food prices, protein supplements and/or high protein diets are financial investments without sufficient return.

The most hotly debated issue today among those who worship strength is the use of androgens, a major male hormone. There is no question that supplementary androgens can produce significant weight gains in athletes. However, the question of whether they lead to the spring of untapped strength is not clear. At last count, I found the medical literature nearly split on the topic—half stating androgens do yield significant increases in muscular strength, and half contesting this proposition. All this may be academic, for it seems only a matter of time until androgens will be banned from most major athletic activities. Their use can be monitored by a very sensitive urine or blood test. Most medical authorities believe they should be outlawed since a growing body of literature has documented serious metabolic and blood pressure changes as the result of androgen use.

For the athlete desiring to gain weight, the most logical method to follow is to increase calorie consumption (with most of the increase being in carbohydrates). Fats have a pronounced satiety effect, so even though on a per weight basis they contain the highest number of calories, it is unusual to be able to gain weight on a high-fat diet. As I mentioned before, protein is expensive and ultimately broken down to sugar fragments. Moreover, recent evidence points to some of the minor breakdown products of protein as direct inhibitors on brain and muscle function. This lethargy and depression in function is transient, but can interfere with an active training program. So if you must, increase the calories with the carbohydrates!

WEIGHT AND HEALTH

By way of concluding this article let me reiterate my previous contention; weight loss is usually beneficial to one's health. Weight gain rarely is! Except for the actual deficiency disorders (due to vitamin- or mineral-poor diets), I know of no disease caused or accelerated by being skinny. Yet the other side of the coin is shocking. If you are 10% over life-insurance weight for your height, you risk developing high blood pressure at two times the normal rate, diabetes at three times, and gall bladder disease at five times. Long-term followup studies of weightlifters and football players have shown that they have a below-normal life expectancy, whereas studies of cyclists, cross-country skiers and oarsmen found significant increases in life expectancy. It is my position that sports should be healthy; in that sense, thin is more than just "in" with the fashion world—it is good sportsmanship.

The sports where weight is an advantage are few, and college football is one of them. But there's healthy and unhealthy weight. Professional football players, it's been discovered, often have a healthier body fat index than slimmer athletes in non-contact sports. (Joe Melena Photo)

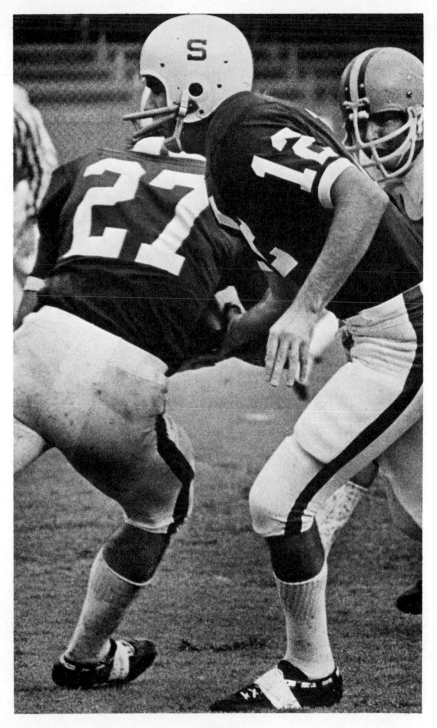

4

The
Last Suppers

The way runners eat before races, you'd think they were worried about dying of malnutrition after 50 meters.

—Arthur Lydiard

The pre-event meal pictured by Arthur Lydiard, a coach of Olympic-winning runners in both New Zealand and Finland, involves as much ritual and superstition as nutrition. In this "last supper" scene, runners are no worse than any other athletes.

The team members and their coaches sit down together. They're all frightened and preoccupied. Conversation is disjointed. Humor is forced. The event is four hours away. Never mind that it's two o'clock in the afternoon. The meal must be four hours before the event.

Everyone eats the same things—a small portion of meat "for strength," toast with honey for "quick energy," tea with more honey to "keep you awake." Never mind that the athletes don't like tea and their nerves already are tearing at their guts. It's critical that they eat this way now.

It's critical, anyway, if the last meal calms the athlete and makes him think he's gaining some slight edge here. But nutritionally, the meal does next to nothing. Nothing positive, that is. There is no record of any athlete fainting from malnutrition during the last lap of a mile race, the last set of a tennis match or the last quarter of a football game. But no one has to look very far to see evidence of nausea, vomiting, stomach cramps or diarrhea caused by combining eating and running.

The bias in this chapter, if not the entire book, is toward running. This isn't only because most of the writers are runners. The best research on athletic diet is coming from this sport—a

-68-

simple sport which is easily studied. Since most strenuous sports involve some running, and few are more strenuous than running itself, the lessons from it have obvious application elsewhere.

Runners are beginning to wake up to several facts about diet in the pre-race period. First, that it may bring as many problems as benefits. Second, they're better off eating nothing than too much. Third, food is a fuel which at best extends their mileage only slightly.

The book *The Runner's Diet* notes, "Food and drink aren't ends but beginnings. They are the fuel that powers training, which in turn is the basis for racing. Minimum amounts and types of food and drink are needed before the process can begin—before health, strength and energy are adequate. But once these minimums are met and running is underway, nutrition offers no substitute for work and no shortcut to success. It merely promotes work and opens the way to success."

The editor adds, "No runner ever got anywhere just by eating. Once runners realize this, they are better able to see what nutrition can offer them. It offers quite a lot, actually.

Unfortunately for anyone hoping to get a last-minute boost before competition (and, in fact, before any unusual physical effort), it's too late to change what is or isn't in the fuel tank. That can only be done slowly, over weeks and months. The last supper does have a direct influence on performance. But more often than not it's a negative one.

ELIMINATE THE NEGATIVE

The entire system is on alert. It wants to explode into action with strength and speed, or to ration effort over a long haul. Either way, the juices are flowing to the extremities. They have no time to waste on the passive work of breaking down food. Take in food immediately before this kind of exertion, and what happens? It sits in a heavy, undigested lump, or is pushed out of one end or the other.

Whatever an athlete eats in the last hours before competition, he won't get much good from it. He can get a lot of trouble, though, and the trouble happens at the worst possible time—when tension or fatigue are peaking.

A basketball player throws up his expensive training-table meal as he leaves the locker room. A cross-country skier doubles over, clutching a knifing pain at his beltline. A race walker pulls out of the race and into the bushes for an emergency pit-stop. All these symptoms can be traced back to the pre-event meal. Considering the alternatives, it might have been better to start with a hungry feeling.

The easiest way an athlete can use diet to his advantage is to eliminate the negatives. There are two basic rules to this:

o *Don't eat the wrong things at the wrong times.*

o *Don't eat too much too late.*

The pre-event hours are no time to experiment with strange foods. Certain stomachs are overly sensitive to certain foods, and tension and stress compound the sensitivity.

On the accompanying page, Dr. George Sheehan, medical editor of *Runner's World* magazine, lists do's and don't's of pre-exercise eating. He summarizes his thoughts with this advice, "I think you shouldn't deviate significantly from your normal foods the day of the race. Most of us try different pre-race meals instead of sticking to our usual meals and foods we know don't bother us."

Sheehan lists three primary offenders: "Coffee is a stimulant to bowel action and should be avoided (immediately before competition). Milk, for those who don't particularly care for it, is a real troublemaker. In special instances, wheat and grain products can cause diarrhea."

The doctor himself is a competitive runner. He says he has had severe diarrhea only once—"when I took a quart of milk and a quart of orange juice for my pre-race meal!" Once was enough.

Dr. Ernst van Aaken, a German physician and running coach, says healthy humans can carry on for long periods while "living off their own resources." He thinks every ounce of food carried during training and competition merely "increases the system's burden."

Van Aaken advises even ultra-marathoners, runners in races of 30–100 miles, to fast for 12–24 hours before competing. They suffer no ill effects from running this way. Other Europeans have shown that skiers and walkers can hike through the mountains for days at a time on little or no food. If they have enough stored fuel to do this, surely a sprinter, weight lifter, gymnast or similar athlete who competes for seconds can go hungry for a little while, too.

Common Food Intolerances

by Dr. George Sheehan

● **Milk:** Milk, after the second decade of life, is something most Greek Cypriots, Arabs, Ashkenazi Jews and American Negroes should shun. These people from traditionally non-milk-drinking areas (and this includes among others the Bantu, Chinese, Thai, Greenland Eskimo and Peruvian Indian; about 8% of Caucasians also have trouble handling milk) can have bloating, gas and stomach pains after even the small amounts of milk used in cooking. Most people with milk allergy do not drink it anyway through some body intuition. If you have never been much of a milk drinker, I think you should accept this "body wisdom."

● **Grain:** Many men, it appears, cannot live by bread *at all,* much less alone. A distance runner complained to me that every time he entered a long, tough race he came down with severe stomach pain. Sometimes he would have diarrhea and blood as well. He only developed the symptoms after a hard run. He had no known allergies, and even varying his pre-race diet didn't help. He continued to experience pain severe enough to double him up soon after the race was over. He finally reduced his pre-race feeding to bread and milk, but he still had trouble. There, as it turned out, lay the answer.

Bread, or more specifically, gluten—protein found in all grains except corn and rice—was his difficulty. In its full-blown state, the inability to handle gluten is called "sprue," meaning chronic diarrhea. It now appears that some athletes may have sprue. Most don't, but many, when placed under stress, can become symptomatic. When the rat-race pushes them too fast or too far, their bowels let them know.

Gluten is found not only in bread, baked goods and cereals, but is also hidden in soups and gravies, ice cream, mayonnaise and even beer and ale.

● **Coffee:** It causes hyperacidity and stomach spasms in some people, and also creates spasms in people with sensitive or irritable colons. It is a stimulant to bowel action.

- **Highly Allergic Foods:** Chocolate, shellfish, strawberries, pork, melon, nuts, citrus fruits, and egg white can cause stomach pains, diarrhea, bloating, rash, itching, headaches, nasal stuffiness and other symptoms.

- **Excessive Roughage:** Athletes with spastic colons have trouble with raw fruit, raw vegetables, nuts, corn, baked beans, cabbage, etc., which can cause gas, bloating, pain and thin, pencil-like stools.

THE ENERGY CRISIS

For the generations growing up thinking power flows from a light switch and an accelerator pedal, the "energy crisis" of the 1970's may seem new. But any athlete whose event lasts more than a few minutes knows better. The real energy crisis is as old as man, and it has nothing to do with electricity and gasoline. It involves his own fuel. Where to get it? How to use it?

The way man eats and the energy he gets from his food shape the pattern of his life. Food has traditionally set man's limits. The coming of the wheel and the engine have seemed to extend the limits. But when man gets back under his own power, the old rules still apply. They apply most dramatically to athletes who are testing their limits.

The rest of this chapter is meant for endurance athletes—people who move continuously for several minutes to several hours. They're limited not so much by speed, strength or skill as by the amount of energy they have available. When it runs low, they slow down or stop, like a car running out of gas.

Food and drink are the only available fuel sources beyond the air they breathe. But it doesn't follow that athletes who eat the most will endure the longest. Energy is stored by eating and training in the right amounts for the individual, at the right times. It can be stored to incredible degrees.

An American runner, Park Barner, makes a practice of not eating for 24 hours before his races. He began doing this in 1972, before the 52-mile London-to-Brighton race in England. Park improved his best time there by a half hour. The estimated energy cost of such a run is more than 5000 calories. Barner drew them all from his reserves, not from any last-day or en-route snacks.

In 1964, a team of Swedish walkers hiked for 10 days, covering 300 miles. They ate nothing during that time, lost an average of 15 pounds of stored energy, and were none the worse for wear after the trip.

Eminent Swedish physiologist Per-Olof Astrand tells of a three-day cross-country tour of his, in which he covered about 40 miles each day: "The calculated caloric cost was a total of some 18,000 calories. Only 1000 calories were supplied. These came almost exclusively in the form of carbohydrate. Some 14,000–15,000 calories were probably from fat stored in the body."

Dr. Astrand makes two points about energy:

1. Protein foods (meat, fish, poultry, eggs, etc.) play no immediate part in the energy production of exercising athletes.

2. Their energy comes from a mixture of glycogen (a product of carbohydrate foods—cereals, sugars, etc.) and fat. The percentage of each depends on the level of effort. The more violent the exercise, the higher the percentage of glycogen being burned, and vice versa.

Astrand says, "Combustion of protein [is] no higher during heavy exercise than during rest. In one experiment, we compared cross-country skiers who raced 20–50 miles in one day with resting athletes used as controls. There was no noticeable difference in the amount of protein used."

However, he notes, "The utilization of carbohydrate depends on the oxygen supplied to the working muscles. The more inadequate the oxygen supply (anaerobic exercise), the higher the carbohydrate utilization."

Briefly stated, fat is more prevalent than glycogen in the body's storehouses, and fat is the best fuel for low-level work. Glycogen is limited in supply, but carries the major energy-producing burden during high-intensity effort. What does this mean to the athlete immediately before a big test?

Eat little protein? Yes. Dr. Astrand says, "There seems no doubt that it is proper to exclude protein from consideration as a fuel for working muscles."

Eat lots of carbohydrates? Possibly. In certain types of events, the benefit of "carbohydrate-loading" is significant. We'll get to this in the next section.

Eat lots of fat? No. The fat that becomes energy during exercise is fat already stored inside the body. As Dr. Joan Ullyot points out later, there's a great difference between "trained-on" and "eaten-on" fat.

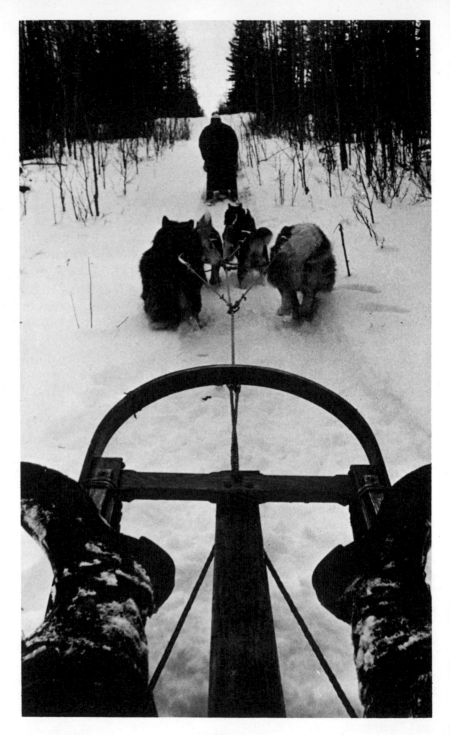

CARBOHYDRATE-LOADING

"For years," said Paul Slovic, "discussions about the influence of diet upon athletic performance tended to emphasize the benefits of protein and vitamins. However, few if any of the enthusiastic claims for these substances have been confirmed by scientific tests. Thus, it was rather surprising when highly respected Swedish physiologists described a diet whose proven effects on endurance surpassed even the wildest claims of health-food hucksters."

Slovic, a scientist with the Oregon Research Institute in Eugene, had just completed a study which told exactly how many minutes this diet could shave from a marathon runner's time. The Swedish diet was called "glycogen super-compensation" by scientific types and "carbohydrate-loading" by laymen. It had been popular among long distance runners since the late 1960's.

The Swedes had learned that (1) depleting muscle glycogen, (2) keeping the level down with a low-carbohydrate/high protein diet, then (3) shifting the balance to high carbohydrate intake did wonders for runners' energy. Muscle glycogen levels soared 100% above normal. This meant individuals could hold fatigue at bay for longer than usual periods.

In long races, where runners often run down like clocks in the late miles, this diet quickly won converts. The usual regimen was a "depletion" run one week before the race, then three high-protein days, then three high-carbohydrate days.

Swedish physiologists Karlsson and Saltin applied this routine in a test with 10 distance runners. They ran two races each—30 kilometers (18.7 miles) three weeks apart. Before one race, they ate normally. Before the other, they "loaded." Times under loaded conditions were 7.7 minutes faster than with normal diets.

This group was small, though, and Paul Slovic wanted results on a bigger scale. So he questioned runners at the 1974 Trail's End marathon, and 181 of them responded. Of these, 98 were non-loaders, 27 partial loaders (increased carbohydrate intake but didn't follow the usual depletion sequence) and 56 were full-loaders.

This dogsled racer is taking it easy now, but he'll be up and running after his breather, using up carbohydrates as working energy and for protection from the cold. (Bill Herriot Photo)

"On the average," Slovic wrote, "the glycogen-loaders finished considerably faster than non-loaders (2:57 vs. 3:23). However, the loaders also trained harder, had more experience with marathoning and were somewhat faster in the mile. These factors, rather than diet, may have determined their superior performance."

Slovic used complex statistical methods to take these factors into account, coming up with formulas which accurately predicted each runner's potential in the race. On this basis, the loaders enjoyed a 6–11½-minute advantage over non-loaders. Carbohydrate-loading apparently had improved marathon times by that much.

Slovic said, "Despite marked differences between the design of this study and that of Karlsson and Saltin, the 6–11½-minute improvement is close to their 7.7-minute effect over 30 kilometers. Another similarity between the two studies is that diet has made little or no difference over the first half of the run, but was associated with marked changes in performance over the last quarter of the course." Loaders, as a group, were able to hold their pace while non-loaders slowed markedly.

Those are the advantages of carbohydrate-loading. In the accompanying article, Dr. Ben Londeree, an exercise physiologist at the University of Missouri, lists the techniques. But what about the limitations?

The most obvious one is that it only works in events lasting 30-60 minutes or more. Also, little is known about its effects outside of running, though it would seem to be useful in bicycling, cross-country skiing, race walking and similar endurance sports.

Another problem with the standard routine (three days low-carbohydrate, three days high) has been to survive the first three days. Athletes feel miserable during that period. They're tired and irritable from low blood sugar. Now physiologists are telling them they can forget the bad days.

Dr. Bob Fitts, a US road running champion: "The final level of muscle glycogen super-compensation reached is not affected by the low-carbohydrate phase of the diet. The main purpose of this phase is to lengthen the amount of time between the depletion run and the race . . . I avoid the potential dangers of this phase by taking my long run on Tuesday, followed by a high-carbohydrate diet Tuesday night through Friday, with the race on Saturday morning."

Dr. David Costill, one of America's leading athletic researchers, agrees that the front end of the diet "is not all that important." He says a long run followed immediately by several high-carbohydrate days gives athletes the same peaks in their races without valleys earlier in the week.

Principles of Loading

by Dr. Ben Londeree

1. During prolonged heavy exercise, the carbohydrate stores are gradually depleted. Energy for exercise is derived almost entirely from fats and carbohydrates. Whereas the supply of fats is virtually inexhaustible, carbohydrates, due to volume requirements, are stored in limited quantities.

2. Depletion of carbohydrates leaves only fats available for energy, with the result that the intensity of activity must be reduced considerably (1-3 minutes per mile). Optimal performance requires that the runner avoid depletion during competition.

3. The rate of glycogen depletion is a function of the relative intensity (percent of maximal oxygen consumption). Below an intensity representing 50% of maximal oxygen consumption, about 50% of the energy is derived from fat. At higher intensities, an increasing proportion of the energy is obtained from carbohydrates. This means that glycogen depletion can be delayed by reducing the speed.

4. The time to exhaustion and glycogen depletion is directly related to the initial concentration of glycogen in the muscles. In other words, with higher beginning muscle glycogen levels, an individual can work at a particular intensity of exercise for a longer period of time.

5. In order to bring about glycogen super-compensation, the body first must be stimulated to synthesize extra glycogen-storing enzyme through depletion of the present supply of glycogen. A high-carbohydrate diet without prior glycogen depletion will not produce super-compensation.

6. Whereas liver glycogen is readily depleted by starvation, a low-carbohydrate diet and/or prolonged exercise, the only way to deplete muscle glycogen is through exercise. Carbohydrate can not escape once inside of a muscle fiber.

7. Depletion of muscle glycogen stores occurs only in the active muscle fibers. Consequently, a significant amount of the

depletion activity must be identical with the activity for which the individual is preparing.

8. The greater the glycogen depletion, the greater the stimulation for the synthesis of glycogen-storing enzyme will be. This, in turn, will increase the potential for super-compensation.

9. The longer the depletion is maintained, the greater the stimulation for the synthesis of glycogen-storing enzyme will be. As above, this increases the potential for super-compensation.

10. Depletion can be maintained with a low-carbohydrate diet and continued training. In fact, such an approach will make it less necessary for complete initial depletion via exhaustive exercise and thereby reduce the risk of incurring fatigue injuries.

11. A small amount of carbohydrates (about 60 grams per day) is essential during the depletion phase for adequate functioning of several important systems in the body, e.g., the nervous system, red blood cells and kidneys.

12. Before commencing the high-carbohydrate diet, redeplete through appropriate physical activity. This is to make sure that you are depleting as much as possible and probably will require only 5–10 miles, depending upon the carbohydrate content of your diet since the previous depletion run. If you have not used the low-carbohydrate diet, then this depletion run must be much longer (15-20 miles). This latter approach, of course, exposes the individual to an injury very close to the time of competition.

13. Glycogen super-compensation (following depletion) will occur only to the extent that carbohydrates are made available in the diet. The greater the percent of carbohydrates in the diet, the greater the super-compensation will be. Adequate proteins (2-3 ounces per day), minerals, vitamins and lots of water should be included in the diet also.

14. *Do not overeat* when on the high-carbohydrate diet. Although you will need a positive caloric balance in order to store energy in the form of glycogen, the reduced activity will more than take care of this if you eat your normal amount of food. The important point is to increase the dietary carbohydrate percent.

15. Drink a large excess of fluids while on the high-carbohydrate diet. About 3–4 grams of water are stored with every gram of glycogen. If an inadequate supply of water is drunk, the extra water is withdrawn from other body sources and a relative dehydration will occur. It is not uncommon for infections to result from such dehydration. A good indicator of proper water intake is clear urine. An amber urine means that you need more water.

16. Activity will tend to reduce super-compensation and should be avoided while on the high-carbohydrate diet. Stay off of your feet as much as possible.

17. Once super-compensation occurs, the excess glycogen-storing enzyme is inactivated and the muscles will tend to burn off the excess glycogen during normal activities. Therefore, timing of the peak super-compensation is rather critical and varies among individuals—typically 2–4 days on the high-carbohydrate diet. The time will depend on individual genetic differences and will tend to be shorter for those persons who regularly deplete and super-compensate during their normal training and diet regime. Some symptoms that the peak super-compensation has passed include: bloated feeling, loose bowels and excessive urination.

18. Reduce the quantity of carbohydrates as well as other foods in the diet during the several hours before the event. There is evidence that a large amount of carbohydrates at this time may impair performance.

19. It is not necessary to fully super-compensate for all competitions. For short activities, it probably would be beneficial to increase the percent of carbohydrates in the diet for one or two days only for the purpose of ensuring that glycogen stores are not low. For events lasting 30–60 minutes, moderate super-compensation would suffice (e.g., 10-mile run 48 hours before competition followed by a high-carbohydrate diet and rest). For longer periods of competition, moderate super-compensation would be beneficial, but utilization of the full protocol would produce better results.

20. If, after weighing all the pros and cons, you decide to super-compensate, try it in stages during your training. For example, start with a long run followed by a high-carbohydrate diet (start with principle 12). Keep a detailed log of what you do and what happens. If satisfied, then try the entire series (depletion, low-carbohydrate diet, redepletion, high-carbohydrate diet) but stay on the low-carbohydrate diet only for one day. If there are no adverse effects, then extend the low-carbohydrate diet gradually to a maximum of three to four days. Do not take short-cuts. Remember, you are playing with biochemical dynamite.

FAT: THE BEST FUEL

Americans in general, American athletes in particular, have a hang-up about fat. Fatness and fitness don't go together, they say. They want to be fit. Therefore, fat is a dirty word.

But this isn't always so. In energy terms, it's one of the athlete's two best friends. And since glycogen can't be stored in the body to any large degree, fat is the most important of the two for certain activities.

Dr. Joan Ullyot, a physiology researcher and sub-three-hour marathon runner, says, "In the American and Scandinavian preoccupation with glycogen, the important role of fat has been overlooked. Fat in general is regarded as so much dead weight to carry about. Excess 'depot fat' acquired by overeating is just that. However, much of the body's fat—especially that stored by trained long distance runners—is highly active metabolically and serves as a superior fuel for endurance performance."

Dr. Ullyot explains that this kind of fat "has a much higher energy yield per gram than glycogen (7:1 ratio), is easily stored in the various nooks and crannies of the body, and in fact is preferentially—almost exclusively—burned by migrating birds and other species that must cover long distances. The principal endurance muscle of the human body—the heart—also burns fat in preference to other substrates."

The ratio of fat to carbohydrate in the fuel mixture increases as work becomes longer and slower in nature. Manipulations of diet, type and amount of exercise can increase the effectiveness of the fat-burning system. German Dr. Ernst van Aaken says the main benefit of pre-exercise fasting is to teach the body to "live off its own resources," the main one of which is stored fat.

Dr. Ullyot notes that an athlete's training influences the amount of fat stored within muscle tissue. "A Swiss researcher named Howald did muscle biopsies of well-trained 100-kilometer (62-mile) runners and found an average of 22.3% fat mixed in with

"Fat is a dirty word" in steeplechasing—but researchers have found there's a big difference between "gut fat" and fat stored in the muscles for energy. (John Marconi Photo)

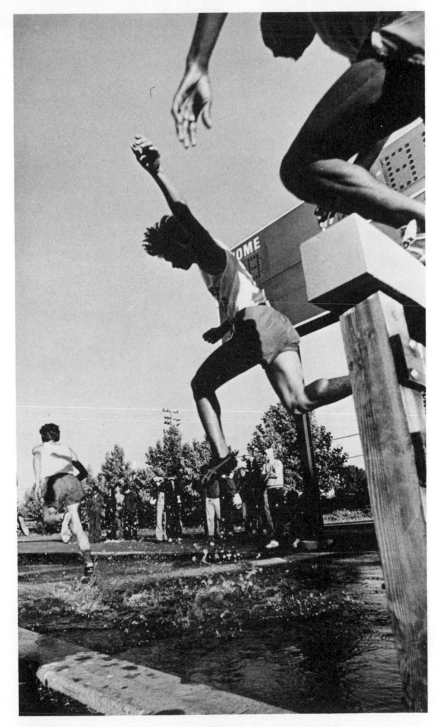

lean muscle. This compared to about 10% in untrained men and in lean runners trained over shorter distances."

But before stocking up on cream and butter, and gaining 15 pounds of fat, read on. Dr. Ullyot points out that fat *within* muscle shouldn't be confused with percentages of total body fat. The latter is quite low in all successful endurance athletes. The 100-kilometer athletes increased their muscular fat through long distance training over many years, not with fat-laden diets.

The doctor says, "The distinction between active, 'trained-on' fat and passive, 'eaten-on' fat is very important. Only the former is useful. Otherwise, the best eater would be the best runner."

5

The Need to Drink

"The 10-mile race in North Carolina was a summer lark for Nelson Hedley. He had let his condition drop off since the track season, but the long race picked up his interest. The temperature was 93. Humidity was high. At five miles, Hedley became dizzy and started to weave. A mile later, he collapsed. He was hospitalized with heat stroke. Examinations revealed he had suffered brain and kidney damage. A week after the race, Hedley died. He was 16." —1973 Marathon Handbook

There aren't many life and death situations in the area of athletic nutrition. No one has been known to starve during an event. But they have literally died of dehydration. Young Nelson Hedley was one of the victims.

The setting was a tragically familiar one. An out-of-shape athlete overreaching his abilities. A hot, humid day. Inadequate fluid replacement (in this case, none at all). As Hedley became dehydrated, his body temperature soared. It probably peaked at 105–110 degrees when he suffered his heat stroke.

The same thing happens each fall to a dozen or more football players. They return to practice less than fit. They practice in the armor of their sport under the broiling sun. They don't take enough timeouts to drink. And we read about their heat strokes in the newspapers.

Long distance runners and football players, athletes at opposite ends of the sports spectrum in terms of body types, share a particular susceptibility to problems of the heat—runners because they're running so long, football players because they wear so much. They both sweat huge amounts, and don't or can't replace the fluids adequately.

The body's water-chemical balance is delicate. Sweat losses as small as two or three pounds may affect performance. Double that figure and the losses may affect health itself. An athlete can sweat away dangerous amounts in less than an hour. Nelson Hedley's heat stroke, for instance, occurred less than 45 minutes into his run.

Of course, not everyone who gets deeply into sweat-debt dies from it. Some athletes are merely permanently injured. Gary Castner, a runner from Florida, collapsed after a marathon. He says, "I was taken to a hospital suffering from dehydration and what was later diagnosed as a stroke. It was a slight stroke, and as a result I lost the vision to the left of center in both of my eyes—permanently."

Even if athletes are lucky and don't get hurt by dehydration, the effects (elevated pulse, dizziness, nausea, etc.) can keep them from doing their best in training and·competition. Knowing these facts about the relationship of heat and drinking, it's hard to understand why athletes aren't allowed—either through superstition or legislation—to drink whenever and whatever they want.

Some football coaches still withhold water from their athletes, warning them that "it will give you stomach cramps." (That may occasionally be true, but the alternative is far more serious.) Long distance runners are prevented by international rules from drinking as early or as often as they should. (By the time they get their first legal drink—at seven miles—it may already be too late to do any good.)

Anyone who restricts his athletes' water supply is playing a foolish game.

SWEATING AWAY FITNESS

Jockeys do it. Wrestlers do it. Even overweight joggers do it. But that doesn't mean it's the right thing to do. It's hard enough keeping an adequate fluid supply without intentionally sweating it away inside a steam cabinet or under layers of rubberized clothing.

Quick sweating gives a phony kind of weight loss. To lose a pound of fat requires running for 30–40 miles. A pound of sweat disappears 10 times faster. But the quick loss doesn't stay lost. Two glasses of water put it right back on.

While these water-weight losses are temporary, they're still important to athletes. And the significant effects are negative ones, ranging from impaired performance to heat collapse. Here, in simplest terms, is what happens: a pint of sweat weighs about a pound, and an athlete can be down by about a quart before noticing that anything is wrong. As the deficit grows, the body temperature goes up proportionately, pushing toward a critical level.

Dr. C.H. Wyndham, a South African, has done extensive research involving heat responses. Reporting results of his studies, he said, "Up to a water deficit of about 3%, body temperature varied between about 101 and 102 degrees (F). But with an increase in the water deficit above 3%, rectal temperature increased in proportion to the extent of the water deficit." (See accompanying chart for the 3% figures.)

American physiologist Dr. David Costill has measured sweat losses as great as 10% in marathon runners, and rectal temperatures as high as 105 degrees. Drinking immediately before and during runs won't completely eliminate these conditions, but can replace enough of the lost fluid and cool the temperatures to a degree where exercise is at least safe.

Dr. Costill describes his testing: "In the laboratory, we conducted a series of three two-hour runs, at six minutes per mile (20 miles on the treadmill). During two of the runs, the subjects were fed a total of 4.5 pounds of water or Gatorade. One of the runs was performed without fluid replacement."

THREE PERCENT WEIGHT LOSS

Pre-Exercise	Post-Exercise*	Pre-Exercise	Post-Exercise*
100 lbs.	97 lbs.	150 lbs.	145 lbs.
105 lbs.	102 lbs.	155 lbs.	150 lbs.
110 lbs.	107 lbs.	160 lbs.	155 lbs.
115 lbs.	112 lbs.	165 lbs.	160 lbs.
120 lbs.	116 lbs.	170 lbs.	165 lbs.
125 lbs.	121 lbs.	175 lbs.	170 lbs.
130 lbs.	126 lbs.	180 lbs.	175 lbs.
135 lbs.	131 lbs.	185 lbs.	180 lbs.
140 lbs.	136 lbs.	190 lbs.	184 lbs.
145 lbs.	141 lbs.	195 lbs.	189 lbs.

*Post-exercise weights including water replaced during the training or competition, but with no drinks after finishing.

After the two runs with drinks, the athletes' stomachs were pumped to see what had become of their liquid intake. "We found," Costill says, "that only about 81% of the 0.54 gallons ingested had actually been absorbed from the stomach. We have estimated that a runner will lose about 3.7 pounds per hour, but he can only remove about 1.8 pounds of water from his stomach in the same period. That means that regardless of how much a runner drinks, it will be impossible for him to keep up with the weight being lost by sweating."

Despite this net loss, Costill found evidence that drinking on the run was helping these athletes. Amby Burfoot, the 1968 Boston marathon champion, registered an internal temperature of 105.5 when he ran without drinking, but dropped to 103.6 when he drank. The doctor says, "Since a body temperature above 104.5 can cause extreme distress and possible collapse, this cooling quality of ingested fluids could be of paramount value on a warm day."

Dr. Costill says athletes tend to let the sensation of thirst set their drinking habits, and thirst sometimes lies about their true needs. "Man generally relies on his thirst to control body fluid balance," he says. "Unfortunately, this mechanism is far from accurate. In laboratory tests that required about eight pounds of sweat loss, we found that thirst was temporarily satisfied by drinking as little as one pound of water."

After a sweat loss this large, it may take days to redress the balance. Chronic dehydration may result from repeated heavy fluid drains and inadequate replacement. The best way to guard against this, according to Costill, is to check your weight each morning before breakfast. If you're down two or three pounds from the day before, don't kid yourself that you've lost fat which you can do without. It doesn't happen that fast. You're low on liquid and can't afford that kind of loss.

WHEN WATER ISN'T ENOUGH

Sweat is mostly water, of course, but it is more than that. It has various dissolved chemicals in it, too—notably sodium chloride and potassium—and drinking plain water won't replace them. So while water is good for putting down the thirst of sports, mixed drinks with salt and potassium (and perhaps sweeteners) added are even better.

Dr. George Sheehan, author of the *Encyclopedia of Athletic Medicine,* has looked at the dehydration problem from the points of view of both the athlete and physician. He writes, "There is now general agreement about what to do: fluids, fluids and more fluids. This is the first priority. The amounts of fluid lost and therefore needing to be replaced can be astounding. The second priority is sodium chloride, then potassium. These electrolytes, as they are called, are found in the commercial 'Ade' drinks, though sometimes in insufficient quantity." He warns, however, that "alone, salt and potassium are nothing. In fact, salt without water does more harm than good."

Certain natural and manufactured solutions revive hot and thirsty athletes faster than water, if the chemicals and the water are in sweat-like proportions. The salt-potassium balance is particularly important.

The magazine *Medical Times* reports, "The need for potassium is especially applicable when salt is being given, for it has been found in hot climates that increased salt intake enhances potassium excretion. Also, a large series of heat stroke cases reviewed has shown that potassium depletion in the serum was present in a majority of cases."

Medical Times researchers studied the properties of several drinks—including the commercial preparations Gatorade, Sportade and Half-Time Punch. All three had similar salt content—about the same as found in a glass of whole milk. Potassium was highest in Sportade—five to ten times more than in Gatorade or Half-Time Punch, but only half the potassium level of whole milk or orange juice.

Dr. Martin Eisman concluded that these three mixed drinks are inadequate to cope with the fluid loss of an athlete who isn't adapted to the heat, but that they work reasonably well for an acclimatized individual. The amounts of salt and potassium lost through sweating decrease as athletes adapt to heat.

Of the "synthetic sweat" drinks analyzed, Dr. Sheehan rates Sportade first, Half-Time Punch second and Gatorade a distant third. But he thinks another solution, E.R.G. (Electrolyte Replacement with Glucose) runs well ahead of these competitors. Sheehan adds, "Orange juice with a weak salt solution may be a good homemade substitute."

Dr. Eisman opts for tomato juice with a water chaser. He says equal volumes of the two drinks provide athletes with more than adequate amounts of salt and potassium. Tomato juice, how-

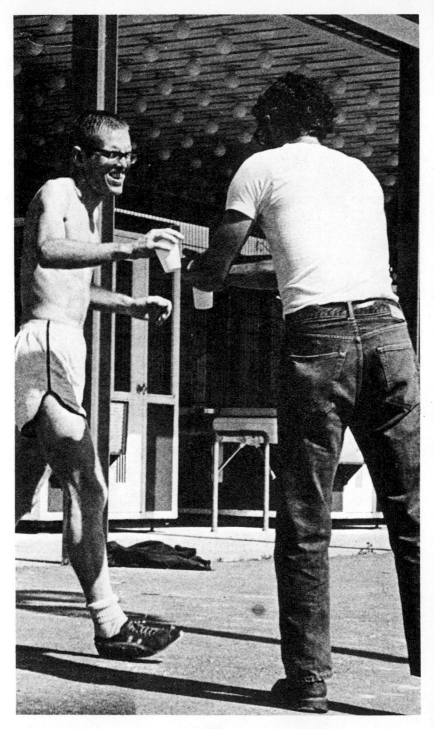

ever, doesn't taste too good—especially in the middle of a hard race or game. Also, tomato juice doesn't give the same energy boost as sweeter drinks.

Peter van Handel of the Human Performance Laboratory, Ball State University, says most athletes "drink the various commercially available 'Ades' or other homemade solutions to provide quick energy. I have seen national caliber endurance athletes take honey on a spoon in an attempt to delay fatigue."

Does it work? Van Handel can't give a simple yes or no. The effectiveness of the sweeteners as energy apparently depends on their concentration in a solution.

"In general," he says, "the more carbohydrate in the drink, the longer it takes the solution to get out of the stomach. The energy available in the drink *cannot* be used until the carbohydrate leaves the stomach and enters the blood from the small intestine.

"Numerous studies have shown that salt solutions leave the stomach very rapidly, and the addition of even small amounts of sugar can drastically slow down the rate of emptying. This slowing delays the movement of water into the circulation."

Van Handel says that in hot weather, "prevention of dehydration and heat stress is of utmost importance. Carbohydrate supplementation is secondary. Therefore, under these conditions the sugar content of the drink should be minimal so that water can rapidly enter the circulating blood." He says the sugar concentration shouldn't exceed 2½%.

Van Handel works at Ball State University with Dr. David Costill, whose work in athletic physiology is known worldwide. Costill's advice for drinking on hot days is this: Drink early and often (he recommends a pint 10 minutes before training or competition, and a half-pint at 10–15 minute intervals during). Don't wait until you feel thirsty, or you'll already be too far in sweat-debt to escape.

Ultramarathoner Ken Young takes in electrolytes and glucose during a 100-mile run in the hot weather of Sacramento, California. Young's brew isn't known, but the enormous internal stresses of this kind of nonstop effort must be eased by the right balance of liquid intake and replacement of minerals lost through sweating. (OMPhoto)

6

The Drug Problem

by Dr. Creig Hoyt

I was reviewing recently the prolific and kaleidoscopic life of the great 20th century man of letters, Aldous Huxley. In so doing I came across a picture of Huxley gazing over a smogless Hollywood; his sublime posture of contemplation and reflection is said to be a result of his being under the influence of mescaline at the time. I reflected that just as the myth of clean air in Los Angeles is ruthlessly refuted by the continual orgy of campers, trucks, and 5000-pound "family" cars plying the southern California freeways, so also is the dream of unlimited potential for mind-expanding drugs currently confronted by the entangled multiple social problems caused by illicit drug usage. The question of drug use by athletes is one still hotly debated by our society, despite the fact that drugs permeate every aspect of our culture.

A recent editorial in a medical journal specializing in sports medicine suggested that it was "our idealism about Corinthian sportsmanship" which compels us to demand that our athletes "be uncontaminated by this distortion of natural life." Whether this thesis emphasizing the Greek ideal of athletic purity is correct is not my main concern in this article. Rather I would like to review our current knowledge of the pharmacology of drugs which athletes might use to improve their level of performance.

The 1974 scandal involving an NFL team whose physician made available enormous quantities of amphetamines for use during competition is only one facet of the question about the proper role of drugs in athletics. Most readers would categorically condemn such a practice. However, what about the use of intra-articular steroids for tennis elbow, anabolic steroids for weightlifters, or even the carbohydrate-loading diet for endurance athletes? These are all questions involving drugs (in the broadest sense of the word). In fact, the use of salt tablets during hot weather athletics must be viewed as a part of the discussion of drugs in athletics. In this article it will be impossible to even survey the entire range of substances which fall under scrutiny as drugs, but I shall discuss several quite different agents, from the lowly aspirin to the major league intoxicants.

AMPHETAMINES

Amphetamines ("speed") are a group of chemicals which have a powerful stimulating effect on the central nervous system as well as a peripheral effect on heart, lungs and blood vessels. The therapeutic indications for these drugs are now quite limited. Indeed, a proposal before the FDA (Food and Drug Administration) would limit their use to the treatment of narcolepsy (a rare disease of sudden attacks of uncontrolled sleep), and a specific pediatric psychiatric disorder (hyperkinetic children).

Currently, the greatest use of amphetamines is in the suppression of appetite for weight reduction. However, although weight loss in dogs is marked when they are given these drugs, sustained weight loss in humans is not significant when clinically accepted doses are utilized. Even less justifiable is the widespread use of these drugs by truck drivers and students to combat fatigue.

The problem is not that the drugs fail to promote a sense of well-being, increased energy and euphoria; it is rather, that repeated use of these drugs induces an early tolerance for them. That is, that one must take larger and larger doses to achieve the same psychological effects. With these larger doses the risk of serious side-effects becomes prominent: psychiatric reactions, seizures, and even sudden death due to cardiac arrhythmias.

However, the essential question for athletes is what improvement in their performance can be attributed to the use of these drugs. Early reports in the 1930's suggested that amphetamines would benefit the athlete by reducing his sense of fatigue. Undoubtedly, the widespread use of these drugs in athletics is the result of whole-hearted acceptance of this thesis. However, after the bicycling drug scandals some 20 years ago, several different European medical centers conducted controlled studies on the performance of various athletes while under the influence of amphetamines. The results were unexpected. Whereas the athletes reported a feeling of running, cycling or swimming more efficiently and powerfully, objective results showed no significant improvement in performance levels while under the influence of amphetamines. Furthermore, many athletes became less coordinated while performing fine skilled motor movements. These same results have been duplicated many times since then.

Scientists are currently in agreement that amphetamines may induce a feeling of improved performance, but actual improvement is the exception. The question must be raised: why are these drugs so widely used by athletes? I think the only answer is that the purely subjective euphoria produced by these compounds is their continuing attraction. The axiom from some professional football circles that "speed makes you mean" needs no comment, and is perhaps a suitable postmortem for a discussion on amphetamines.

LSD, MESCALINE AND HASHISH

These drugs, variously referred to as hallucinogens, psychogenics, or psychomimetics, all have in common the ability to induce visual, auditory and tactile hallucinations as well as gross alterations in mood and normal thought processes. The complete pharmacology of these drugs is not yet established. Frankly, however, their marked alteration of all sensations is of such intensity that they would seem to offer little aid to the serious athlete.

An interesting exception to this statement is that of the Mescacero Apaches in Mexico who still observe an annual peyote ritual. In the spring these Indians run barefoot through the surrounding hills in a 24-hour ritual of peyote consumption, prayers, dancing and endless running. After some American university anthropologists recorded the fact that some of the Indians were able to run up to 75 miles in less than 24 hours, the Mexican government, in a moment of chauvinistic inspiration, decided to enter some of these Indians in the Mexico City Olympics (1968). The results of this experiment, unfortunately, were never obtained. The Mescaceros, who were taken to Mexico City for training, could see no point to running around an oval track with shoes and at short distances like the marathon (26 miles, 385 yards).

Last year an article in *Runner's World* on these Indians, and also a report by the famous British distance runner Bruce Tulloh who visited the area, both concluded that peyote is only used during ceremonial rites. Nonetheless, Mescaceros run 75 to 100 miles without the drug, and it seems their performance is little changed with or without the drug. Yet, the myth continues about the running skills of these fascinating people being assisted by peyote.

Marcia Morey at the US/East Germany meet in 1974. Doping is rare in swimming, despite the hullabaloo over Rick DeMont's elimination at Munich. (Dave Drennan Photo)

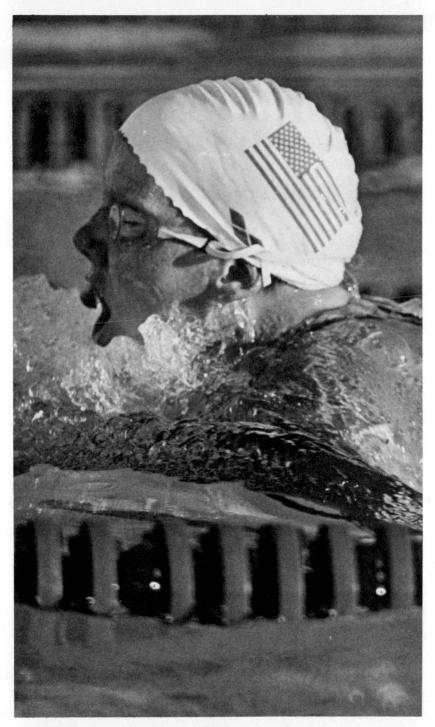

Mescaline and LSD still hold a promising future in the investigation of the nature of schizophrenia and other psychiatric illnesses. The creative potential of these drugs as outlined by Huxley, Alan Watts, and others has not yet been studied in any detailed fashion. The toxicity of these drugs is also incompletely documented. Genetic damage in infants born of LSD-using parents is not a frequent occurence; in fact, recent evidence suggests that it is no more common than random genetic aberrations unrelated to any drug therapy. Reported permanent psychiatric illnesses resulting from the use of these drugs may simply reflect the "normal" psychiatric destiny of those persons drawn to drug excess. Nonetheless, the use of these drugs is on the decline in most areas as a result of the bad reputation they carry within the drug culture. Why the bad reputation? Perhaps science is behind in its documentation of the problems that users know too well. The real discrepancy between subjective and actual performance while under these drugs has been a startling realization for many of the original drug advocates.

On the other hand, the use of hashish in the United States and elsewhere is so widespread in its acceptance that movements to legalize its use seem an inevitability. That many young athletes smoke hashish during their non-competitive hours would appear to be an irrefutable fact. However, the effect that this might have on athletic performance has not been adequately studied. The impression that marijuana's toxicity is much less devastating than alcohol's is a common contention in even standard pharmacology texts. Yet, few well-documented controlled studies have been published to substantiate this belief. The benign nature of the effects of hashish on American users may reflect the fact that long term usage (20 or more years) has not been examined (due to the relatively recent acceptance of this drug), and more important, is the fact that the purity of the "grass" generally available here is so poor that the accumulative dose of the bioactive substance(s) is small. The chronic brain damage documented in the Tangiers hashish pit residents is an eloquent statement refuting the naive assumption that hashish has no serious side-effects.

OPIUM, HEROIN AND MORPHINE

These related drugs are well-known analgesics (pain-killers). They provide dramatic relief for millions of patients each year. However, in addition to their pain-relieving ability, they have a strong euphoria-inducing potential. This aspect of these drugs has led to a global abuse of narcotics. It has recently been reported that some injured football players have received demerol or morphine prior to games in order that they might play without perceiving the pain of their previously existing injuries. I do not doubt the authenticity of these reports, but for most individuals the sedation and lethargy produced by these drugs would be the antithesis of the mood changes required for athletic encounters.

Tolerance to the effect of these narcotics is quickly developed, just as in the case of amphetamines. Indeed, tolerance may be quite marked after only a few experiences with these drugs. Although opium was described in Sumerian texts dating back to 4000 B.C., the mechanism of action of these compounds is only partially understood. It is believed that their primary target organ is the brain and its vital centers (rather than peripheral nerves). In addition to the depression of consciousness produced by these drugs, respirations and heartbeats are decreased. Many of the gothic tales of death resulting from overdoses of these drugs are due to the depression of the brain centers which have to continually trigger respirations. However, all in all, the potential for long term misuse of these drugs by active athletes seems remote. The depressing effects of these compounds are simply too profound to be compatible with quality athletic performances.

ALCOHOL

The detrimental results of alcohol consumption by athletes are multiple. They include: impaired coordination, reduced heat tolerance, decreased maximum oxygen uptake and reduced muscle contractile strength. The world-wide acceptance of self-intoxication with alcohol (even among athletes) is a major public health issue in all countries of the world (except perhaps Red China). Yet, for the serious athlete alcohol can be a disaster at sub-intoxicating doses.

Muscle incoordination can be documented in some individuals after as little as a single beer or highball. In others it may require three drinks in less than 30 minutes to produce similar disabilities. This individual variation in tolerance to alcohol's incoordinating effects is due to both genetic differences (the American indian has a well-documented decreased tolerance to alcohol) and the amount of alcohol usually consumed by the individual (habitual users develop a chemical tolerance by increasing the amount of enzyme available to break down alcohol). It is also true that the more one weighs, the more alcohol one can consume without incoordination troubles. Incoordination may persist for up to 24 hours after drinking alcohol. The slight morning-after tremulousness can be most disastrous to sports requiring fine hand-eye coordination (tennis, golf, etc.).

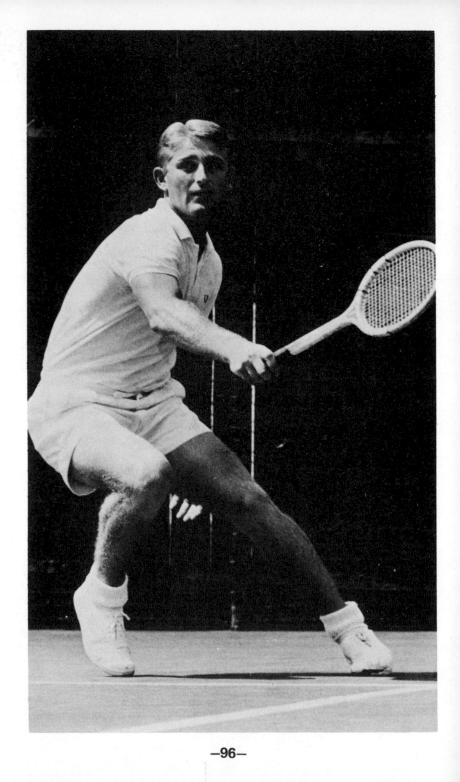

Even more long-lasting is the decreased heat tolerance produced by alcohol. Several studies have shown that a single beer can reduce an athlete's heat tolerance for 24–48 hours. More alarming is the fact that three or more drinks within a single 24–hour period can reduce one's heat tolerance for up to 10 days. This is certainly alcohol's most long-lasting effect (and least well recognized) on athletic performance.

The decrease in aerobic power and muscle contractile strength from alcohol are less dramatic than the two above phenomena. Furthermore, they are short-lived acute effects which should not be noticeable unless one attempts to compete while under the influence of alcohol. The completely devastating picture of permanent physiological changes seen in chronic alcohol abusers need not be outlined here; however, alcohol's social acceptability should not mask its profound alterations in the physiology of even the best-trained athlete.

TOBACCO

With the more militant and relentless cries from the non-smoking public demanding its right to clean air, I know very few people willing to attempt a defense of smoking as anything other than a dirty habit, difficult to break once established. My own position is that tobacco is one of the very few drugs I know without any significant redeeming attribute. The direct effect of cigarette smoking on the incidence of lung cancer, emphysema and bronchitis, and heart attacks is well known. A recent article in a respected British medical journal, *The Lancet*, stressed that it is not only the smoker's health that suffers from tobacco use. In a study in Britain it was shown that children whose parents smoked had two to three times the incidence of pneumonia and bronchitis than children of non-smoking parents. The documented effects of tobacco on the exercising individual are equally shocking.

Tobacco smoke contains 4% carbon monoxide. The affinity of carbon monoxide for hemoglobin (the oxygen-carrying pigment of the blood) is 200–300 times that of oxygen. Thus smokers chemically inhibit the amount of oxygen available to their tissues. A 10–12 cigarette per day smoker will lower his oxygen concentration 5%. This decrease may not be evident at rest, but it will become quite noticeable during almost any exercise. Furthermore,

You can get away with a lot of "social doping" in tennis—smoking, a drink now and then—but it'll keep you from finding your real "outer edges" in performance and vitality.

it may take three to five days after you stop smoking for your body to completely eliminate the carbon monoxide from your bloodstream. Looking at this problem from just a slightly different angle, even the most rigorous training program of a professional endurance athlete can only yield an increase of 10–12% in the maximum oxygen uptake; a pack of cigarettes may reduce the oxygen uptake by seven to ten percent.

In addition, the inhalation of tobacco smoke produces a two- to threefold rise in airway resistance (thus making it difficult to take a deep breath). While this is initially only a transient acute effect, an only slightly less dramatic swelling in the airway (trachea and bronchi) is evident as a permanent defect in the chronic smoker. At rest the pulmonary ventilation may be less than 10 liters per minute; this increase in airway resistance is not noticeable. However, during exercise this airway obstruction may become the primary limiting factor in exercise performance.

STEROIDS

The wonder drugs, steroids, are known to almost every layman. These powerful compounds are the normal hormones produced by our own adrenal glands. Their actions are seemingly endless—on the metabolism of proteins, fats and carbohydrates, on the regulation of water and salt balance, on reducing inflammation, on increasing muscle, kidney and heart function, etc. With only minor chemical alterations the pharmaceutical houses can produce a compound which exerts primarily a single desired effect.

The two major uses of these drugs by athletes have been in regards to their ability to reduce inflammation and to increase muscle bulk (and body weight).

The use of anti-inflammatory steroids may be accomplished by the oral route or by injection. During the last 10 years or so the big business of professional sports has promoted the use of steroid injections into muscles, tendons and joints prior to contests in order to reduce the pain of inflamed tissues. Initially medical opinion was not opposed to this technique; unlike injections of local anaesthetics, steroids do not usually produce complete pain relief. Therefore, it was reasoned that athletes would not be endangered by the total lack of pain which might fail to warn them of a serious injury (this phenomenon is all too often seen in the xylocaine-injected sportsman).

However, as this procedure became more widespread, some alarming results emerged. First, steroid injections prior to, or between contests frequently prolong the average healing time for muscle and tendon injuries. Secondly, non-absorbed residual deposits of these drugs have been found in and around damaged tendons and muscles. Although steroids have not yet fled from the locker room, they are definitely on the decline. Tendon rupture is more common after local steroid treatment than when not used. Recently, an orthopedic surgeon in Los Angeles stressed that steroid injections may actually prolong tennis elbow, not cure it.

The anabolic effect of steroids (weight gain and increase in muscle bulk) is said to be the reason why so many field competitors (discus and shot men particularly) were 25–35 pounds heavier in the 1972 Olympics than in previous competitions. During the Montreal Olympics, it seems unlikely that this will be true again. Last year, Dr. Roger Bannister announced the development of a precise immunofluorescent method for detecting these steroids in the blood or urine (even after several weeks of no drugs). The famous miler, now a renowned neurologist and athletic advisor to Her Majesty, believes the test will be available for international meets within the next year.

The athletic community is still debating the efficacy of anabolic steroids; some studies have suggested that while they may induce weight gain, they do not increase strength. The tide, however, is very much against them. Several eastern European nations have suggested that they will not abide by any restriction of these steroids. Nonetheless, I think they will eventually be banned by most athletic organizations, but it may take the skills of Dr. Kissinger to pacify all the factions involved in what will almost certainly be a nasty dispute.

ASPIRIN AND SOME OTHERS

A comprehensive discussion of our current knowledge of the common analgesics used by athletes for common minor stresses would constitute an article in itself. However, I should like to mention a few recent events which are gradually changing our thinking about these drugs.

Because of the increasing evidence that darvon (propoxyphene) is not totally without addictive potential the FDA is considering restricting more carefully the use of this drug. This would probably cause some uproar, but several studies have indicated that darvon is no better than aspirin as a pain-reliever. Of course, aspirin itself is no longer pictured as a trivial drug. New research dealing with the nature of prostagladins—hormones involved in a multitude of tissue reactions—has begun to delineate the mechanism of action of aspirin. While the benefits of aspirin's inhibition of the clotting process may prove helpful in patients with small strokes, it may

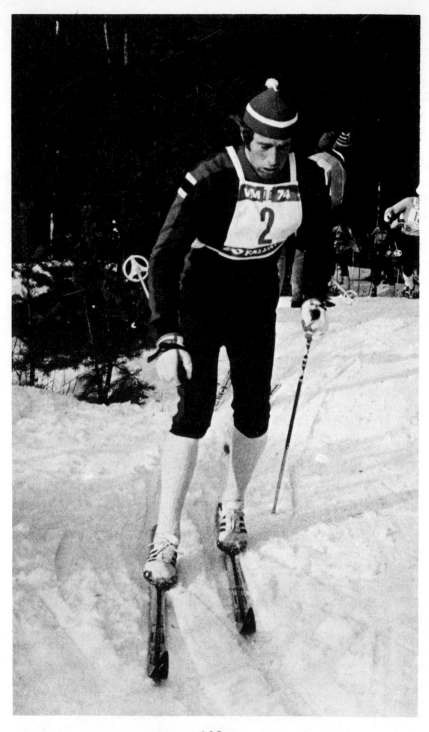

become the very reason that athletes will turn away from the drug. A West German study recently proposed that aspirin may increase small vessel bleeding in muscle and tendon injuries, and is therefore counterproductive in treating these disorders. Furthermore, a great percentage of gastrointestinal bleeds occur within the immediate time following aspirin ingestion.

The above cryptic statements are not meant to imply that darvon, aspirin and other minor analgesics have no legitimate places in sports medicine. However, I think that as the data has been collected on these drugs, their limitations have become considerable.

SUMMARY

Drugs play a definite role in modern medical therapeutics, but their abuse and side effects rival their legitimate value. In a day when 70 million Americans drink alcohol, 90 million smoke tobacco, and the average American medicine cabinet contains 16 prescription medications, I doubt we can seriously construct a case for the majority of Americans adhering to a belief in "naturalness"— life without drugs. Furthermore, I suggest that the public is alarmed only when the less socially accepted drugs are included in the adventures of their sports heroes. Indeed, the bravado with which Dan Jenkins' novel *Semi-Tough* was discussed in even the most reserved circles a few years ago would indicate that most of us not only expect our sports idols to carry on in a drunken, hedonistic fashion—we actually revel in such tales. Nonetheless, I hope the above data have suggested to you that almost any drug may alter your athletic performance, and a healthy skepticism about drugs may benefit your athletic pursuits.

Cross-country ski racing great Magne Myrmo of Norway leads at the 1974 World Championships held in Sweden. Sports like this seem far-removed from the "winning is everything" world of professionalism. Yet the temptations are great and vary in strength with how we define success. (Lennart Strand Photo)

7

The Dietary Revolution

*All people and nations eat too much,
and for this reason are poor performers.*
Paavo Nurmi, 1925

"I'm only 29, but my legs have gone. Can you give me anything that'll buck me up?"

"I'll tell you in a minute. What do you eat?"

The speakers were Raphael Geminiani, famous French professional racing cyclist, and Maurice Messegue, a French nutritionist/herbalist who's advised prominent Europeans ranging from ex-King Farouk of Egypt to Pope John. Messegue put "Gem" on a diet he'd concocted especially for athletes. Geminiani recovered his legs and placed high in the French championships the same year. The reform diet Messegue prescribed consisted of a high proportion of raw vegetables and fruit, whole grains and honey.

Geminiani is just one of many athletes who've experienced the benefits of food reform. Messegue has treated scores of cyclists, including the legendary Fausto Coppi and Luis Ocana, and the results speak for themselves—though Messegue confesses to failure in Coppi's case: the *campionissimo*'s long depression vanished only when he met his wife-to-be.

G.T. Wrench, M.D. is an English physician who has been preoccupied all his professional life with people who show above average health. His story of the Hunza of northeast India was published as an extremely interesting book, *The Wheel of Health*.

Dr. Wrench was impressed by the Hunza's physical performances. He learned of one messenger who traveled on foot 280 miles in seven days, including two traverses of a 15,600-foot pass. This drew no special comment from the Hunzas, who considered it a routine feat. During the British occupation of India the Hunzas were considered the equals of the Sherpas of Nepal for hard mountaineering work and portage. All visitors to the remote land have been impressed by their uniform cheerfulness, pride, energy and freedom from disease.

The Hunza diet is marked by simplicity and moderation: "Nothing before going out in the early morning to the fields; after two or three hours of work, bread, pulses and vegetables with milk; at midday, fresh fruit or dried apricots kneaded with water; in the evening these same foods, with meat on rare occasions." The staples are wheat bread, barley, millet, vegetables, milk, buttermilk, clarified butter, curd cheese and a huge quantity of fruit.

Murray Rose was the youngest triple Olympic gold medalist in history at the time of his swimming successes in the late '50's and early '60's. Contrary to the trend of early retirement in swimming, Murray continued to set records to age 23. Murray never tasted meat in his life and since childhood his diet had been carefully arranged along food-reform principles by his parents. Ian Rose, Murray's father, tells the rationale behind his athlete-son's diet in *Faith, Love, and Seaweed.* Murray got his protein from nuts, cheese, soybeans, legumes, goat's milk, yogurt, brewer's yeast, whole grains, sunflower, millet and sesame seeds. Fruits and vegetables were the principle staples of his diet.

Ian Rose did extensive diet research while arranging his son's nutrition plan, and one of his interesting discoveries was the diet of ancient Greek Olympic champions. Fried and boiled foods were frowned on. Very cold drinks were forbidden, and cakes of barley and wheat were important items.

Rose mentions another famous group of Australian vegetarian diet advocates: milers Herb Elliott and John Landy and their controversial coach, Percy Cerutty. "After Herb Elliott had ripped the mile record to shreds in August 1958," reports Rose, "his breakfast training diet was reported by the New York press to consist of walnuts, diced bananas, dried fruits and raw oats." Both of these early running stars were vegetarians while under Cerutty's guidance.

Larry Lewis was one of the most remarkable athletes ever to live, and he never entered a competition. Larry lived in Phoenix, Arizona in his early childhood and began his running career when the chief of Larry's Indian tribe decided the villagers should run *en masse* up the slopes of Camelback Mountain for exercise. At 107—95 years later—Lewis was still running six miles every morning around San Francisco's Golden Gate Park. He would then walk across the city to work as a waiter at the St. Francis Hotel. In a

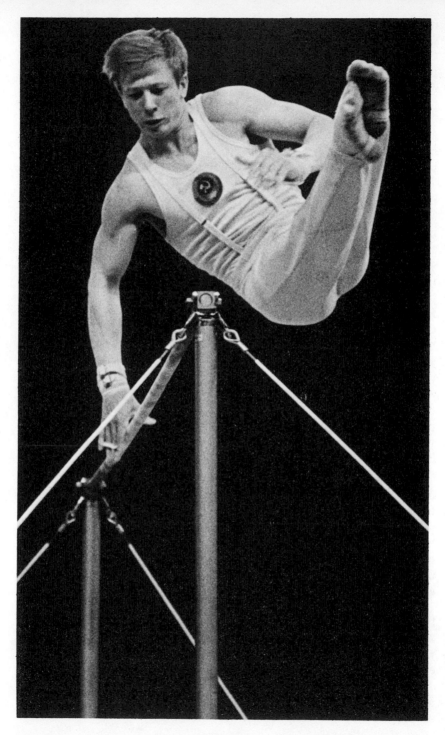

newspaper publicity photo, Lewis was shown at age 105 lifting a 200-pound bank teller two feet off the ground. Larry retired at 104 but found it boring, so went back to work. He ran the 100-yard dash in 17.5 seconds at 102.

Larry Lewis believed in a simple diet. Asked on his 105th birthday how to live long and strong, Larry said, "Do not smoke, drink alcohol, eat fried foods, pastries or white bread; eat only nourishing foods and exercise each day."

Marathon running is full of vegetarians and food-reformers. Eric Ostbye is a legend among marathoners. At over 50 years of age he still runs the 26-mile distance in under 2½ hours, which would qualify him for the US Olympic trials race and places him among his country's top runners. Ostbye switched to a vegetarian diet in 1943. He says diet is the reason he can still run such fast times after more than 20 years of hard training.

John Systad of Norway was a physical wreck in his early teens. His mother, despairing of medical help, put Systad on a vegetarian raw-foods diet. Gradually John worked up to distance running, which he began at 34. Systad eventually won five Norwegian marathon championships, the last at age 43. His diet, refined over the years, is extreme even among reformers: pure orange or grapefruit juice in the morning, herb tea and perhaps an apple for breakfast, fruit at mid-morning and onions, one potato and two slices of whole grain bread for dinner. Hygienists would shudder at those onions, considered toxic, but the obviously low-caloric intake is nothing new among distance runners, who have found they can get by on as little as 1200 calories per day despite long training. (Note that the average marathoner is a featherweight of 120–140 pounds.)

Dutch marathon record holder Aad Steylen ran a world-class 2:19 time at the age of 33. "I am convinced," he said, "that through a particular kind of diet, combined with optimal training, one remains in top form for many years longer, without exhausting the body." Steylen became a vegetarian in 1963. "Since beginning this diet I have had hardly any infectious diseases, tendon, cartilage, joint or muscle injuries. I trace this back to my natural diet, which provides the body with the necessary nutritional and building substances. Nutrients give vital energy. They are just as important as training and are the foundation of health."

The unceasing discipline required of gymnasts like the USSR's Boris Andrianov is incompatible with dietary carelessness. Pride in performance is rooted in care and awareness. (Tony Duffy)

In a careful study during 1906–07 at Yale University (cited in N. Altman's *Eating for Life*) 49 people were divided into groups of meat-eating athletes, vegetarian athletes, and vegetarians doing sedentary work. Dr. Irving Fisher reported the results: only two of 15 meat-eaters were able to hold their arms extended parallel to the ground for more than 15 minutes, while 22 of the vegetarians surpassed that time. None of the "carnivores" reached 30 minutes, while 15 of the vegetarians reached that point, nine exceeding an hour, four going past two hours, and one exceeding three hours. Only three meat-eaters could do more than 325 deep knee bends of the nine who took the test, while 17 of 21 vegetarians got that far. Only one meat-eating athlete could do 1000 knee bends compared with six of the 21 vegetarians. Two vegetarians surpassed 2000; none of the meat-eaters did.

In a comparable study in Brussels, Belgium, vegetarians performed two to three times longer than meat-eaters before complete exhaustion. The "veggies" took only a fifth of the time to recover from the effects of exercise.

A professional strong man of the early '50's known as "The Mighty Young Apollo," who among other feats pulled with his teeth four newspaper delivery trucks, five passenger cars and a double decker bus hitched together, switched to a vegetarian diet with no reported diminution of strength.

Johnny Weissmuller set six world records in swimming after becoming a vegetarian. And Oakland Raiders linebacker Chip Oliver reported playing better after becoming a vegetarian. Portland Trail Blazers basketball star Bill Walton has not eaten meat or fish since 1972. His results speak for themselves.

One of the best-known American vegetarian athletes is comedian Dick Gregory. Gregory originally began fasting as a protest against the Viet Nam war. He has turned a lot of attention since then to the strictly non-political health benefits of diet reform and fasting and recently published an entertaining book about his experiences, *Dick Gregory's Natural Diet for Folks Who Eat: Cookin' With Mother Nature*. Gregory subsisted on fruit juice alone for a very long period, over two years, and ran 10 miles a day for most of that time, during which he also ran the famous Boston marathon. In the summer of 1974 Gregory ran 900 miles in 30 days while living on fruit juice. Thirty miles a day is far more than world-class marathon runners do in training.

The literature of endurance feats performed by diet reformers includes fasting marches, mountain climbing and many other interesting demonstrations. More convincing than these, though, is the amazing record of the English Vegetarian Cycling and Athletics

Club (VCAC). At one time this club held 40% of the national cycling road records. VCAC member Ronald Murgatroid won 15 national events in 1963 and five years later won the best-all-around trophy in the over-40 category, averaging 22.98 mph for the 25-, 50-, 100-mile and 12-hour distances.

The time trialing record of VCAC riders is formidable. Malcolm Amey, a 24-year-old rider who's been a vegetarian for six years, set a new club 100-mile record of 4:13:38 on August 18, 1974. Malcolm's best 25-mile time is a superb 57:11.

Walter Keeler is an amazing VCAC athlete. He's never tasted meat. Now 76, at age 71 the veteran cyclist and race walker covered the 52½-mile London-to-Brighton race walking course just inside the coveted 12-hour standard. The next year he tried to walk 100 miles in 24 hours and had gone 84 miles in 20 hours when he was pulled off the track by officials who doubted his ability to go the remaining 16 miles in four hours.

Sidney H. Ferris set one of the most prestigious records in the cycling books in 1935: two days, six hours and 33 minutes for the 800-mile Lands End-to-John O'Groats course from one end of Britain to the other. Sidney has now been a vegetarian for 49 of his 66 years.

The US is not without its own notable vegetarian cyclists—the biggest "names" among them being Wayne and Dale Stetina. Anyone involved with bike racing knows who Wayne and Dale are, as they are rarely out of the first five places in any race they enter. In a recent *Bike World* interview Dale was asked if the family's vegetarian diet contributed to improved recovery in a hard racing schedule. Stetina said this was true, and that it also contributed to a long career in athletics: "I don't think there's any doubt about it, especially with the meat today and all the contaminants and toxins in it. With the normal toxins in meat, plus the stuff the animals are fed, I don't believe it's got too much to offer, not for the real endurance rider and for top conditioning."

THE HEALTH RADICALS

by Ian Jackson

Ian Jackson is the editor of Soccer World magazine, and resident researcher/writer on physiology and nutrition at World Publi-

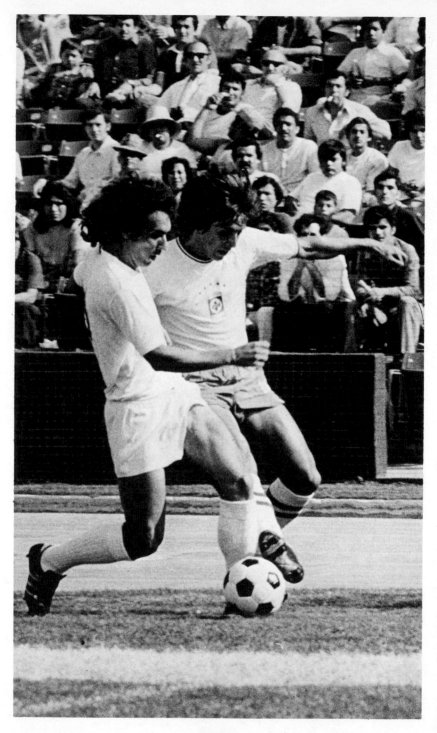

cations. The 30-year-old author of a major forthcoming work on "Yoga for Athletes" has tested his own ideas in the hard light of competition, having run a marathon in 2:33, just three minutes off the Olympic trials qualifying time.

I would never have believed it . . .

"You don't need to eat meat. Sometimes you don't even need food. Many of the top European marathoners are vegetarians who use fasting in their training and racing."

. . . until I tried the European system (the Waerland system) and rewrote some personal records.

I would never have believed it . . .

"You don't have to go to Europe for an ideal health system. The giants of the field are Americans—the *natural hygienists*."

. . . until I got acquainted with the writings of Herbert Shelton, adopted the hygienic system, and rewrote some more personal records.

The ranks of the health reformers are overfull. Bookshelves are loaded with their work: "Be healthy with honey," "Vitamin potencies for new life," "Secret recipes for health and happiness." The gullible public consumes their scribblings by the truckload. Everyone wants to know how many C tablets to take to "prevent" cigarette-caused damage, how much vitamin B to take to compensate for the nightly cocktail, how much E to take to boost failing heart action.

There are no ranks of health radicals. The truth just doesn't sell. No one wants to believe that health is directly related to all factors in lifestyle. They are too fond of their favorite indulgences to take seriously the revolutionary approach. "Stop smoking and drinking, give up the sedentary life? Do you think I'm going to turn into a fitness fanatic? Forget it!"

Most people would like to believe that poor health is misfortune, beyond control like the wind and weather. Most people look upon doctors as their only protection against disease.

A small band of radicals, ridiculed and discounted by the medical profession, has been trying to educate people about their health since the early 1830's. Their message is simple and direct. They do not speak in the mumbo jumbo jargon of "professional" journals. They speak in the language of the people directly to the people. They teach the implications of human physiology for lifestyle. They teach a lifestyle which ensures many years of robust, undoctored health. No wonder the medical profession lays on the scorn.

Medicine treats the sick; hygiene teaches the well. (M.J. Baum Photo)

The first American health radical was an M.D. by the name of Isaac Jennings. In 1822 he began practicing a special brand of medicine. Armed with his own pills, powders and potions, he went out to conquer diseases wherever they lay. Even the most intractable cases responded to his magic. His fame spread far and wide. No other doctors could compete with him.

After about 20 years of astounding success, he revealed his secret. His pills were bread, his powders were colored flour and his potions were colored water. The only "magic" in his methods, the only "secret" to his success, was the body's own powers of self-healing, when given the proper conditions. He ensured that it got those conditions by the very strict and explicit instructions he gave with the "medicine." According to the condition of the patient, he recommended rest, fasting, good diet, pure air, pure water, sunlight and other hygienic factors.

The furor was as wide as his fame. His medical associates were surprised and angry. The same patients who had showered him with gratitude now vilified him for deceiving them. The more intelligent among them offered confused congratulations. "If you can cure our diseases without medicine, then you are the doctor for us."

The more intelligent Americans continued to support him. Yale University awarded him an honorary degree in recognition of the brilliance and originality of his work. When he moved to Oberlin, he was made a trustee of the college, and he served the town as mayor.

Another early American health radical was Sylvester Graham. Through the influence of his devout mother, Graham became a preacher in the Presbyterian church. This led him into temperance work which led to the study of anatomy and physiology, and finally into the practical application of his studies.

He first noticed the importance of diet during a severe cholera epidemic that swept the city of Philadelphia. With the exception of one small group, the populace was dying like flies. This group, a sect of Bible Christians, went among the sick and dying, relieving what suffering they could, in complete and impregnable immunity to the disease.

It was their belief that God had forbidden flesh eating. They ate no meat, fish, eggs, milk or cheese. They used no salt, pepper or condiments of any kind. They drank no tea, coffee or alcohol. Nor did they use tobacco in any form.

Unburdened by the dogmas of medical training, Graham was quick to see the connection between their lifestyle and their resistance to disease. Insights such as these informed his teachings. His lectures were well received by the public and bitterly opposed by the medical profession.

The most controversial of his ideas seem absurdly obvious today, now that we know about vitamins and other nutritional elements. He recommended fresh fruits and vegetables while the doctors of his day spluttered on about their uselessness and even danger as foods. You can still read medical propaganda ridiculing Graham and other pioneers like him. You can read it in today's newspapers.

The list of pioneers is long and illustrious. All of them were courageous and independent thinkers. None of them were afraid to stand against the tide of medical opinion. This band of health radicals, the American hygienists, includes, besides Jennings and Graham, such names as Russell Trall, M.D., Mary Gove, Thomas Nichols, M.D., James Jackson, M.D., Harriet Austin, M.D., Charles Page, M.D., Robert Walter, M.D., Susanna Dodds, M.D. and John Tilden, M.D. Needless to say, none of them were popular with the rest of the medical profession. In their eyes, they were all renegades.

Notice the number of women in the list. The hygienists were practicing women's liberation before it became a household word. At the present time the leader of the movement is Virginia Vetrano. Herbert Shelton is now retired, but he has worked for decades in the care of the sick. He has written volumes of iconoclastic books. He has synthesized and pruned the work of his predecessors, as well as adding much of his own insight. He has just completed, at age 79, a masterpiece of hygienic literature—*Fasting for the Renewal of Life.*

Those who are familiar with the work of the hygienists and know the ridicule they have had to put up with over the years also know that the tide is now turning in their favor. The general public is becoming more and more conscious of the serious questions about even the most common of drugs—aspirin. The thalidomide tragedy put fear into the hearts of pregnant women the world over, and generated justified worries about the use of *any* drugs in pregnancy or at any other time.

And the general public is beginning to believe that the hygienists might be right about exercise, too. They see runners, joggers, cyclists, swimmers and other active people enjoying virtual immunity to disease and boundless energy. They may or may not realize it, but all active athletes are validating hygienic principles and undermining the medical view of health and disease. They are all part of the "witness to fitness" movement.

The most advanced doctors recommend exercise, and they

claim that it is part of "preventive medicine." They should know better. Exercise is by no stretch of the imagination medicine. It is a natural component of health. It is a hygienic factor. When hygienists like Diocletian Lewis tried to get regular exercise included in school programs, the medical profession vehemently opposed it. Now they are trying to claim credit for it, though exercise is no more or less than a normal need of the human organism.

Exercise produces a wonderful change in the body known as as the training effect. When training stresses are regularly applied, the body's own powers bring about this organic adaptation. It is these same powers that heal wounds, fight infections and mend broken bones. The same powers are utilized in both training and healing. In the first case, they transform health to superior health; in the second, they transform impaired health to health. This is why hygienic literature has so much to offer the athlete. It gives detailed, practical advice on how to conserve and develop the body's adaptive energy.

Hygienic measures are designed to supply the body with its basic needs according to its ability to use them. Exercise is a basic need, but it is useless, in fact harmful, when the body is exhausted. The advice not to train when really tired is pure hygienic advice.

Food is a basic need. But it is useless, in fact harmful, when the body cannot use it. In sickness, for instance, the body's resources are mobilized to correct a condition of impaired health. There is no appetite in these conditions. By turning off the appetite, the body is showing that it does not need and cannot use food. In times of sickness, the hygienists recommend fasting.

Waerland, the European hygienist, points out that the work of digesting food is comparable to hard manual labor, like ditch digging. Besides having to secrete quantities of digestive juices, the body must supply energy for the peristaltic movements that push food through the digestive tract.

And yet the medical profession still calls for "plenty of good nourishing food" in times of illness. They still view food as if it were coal for the furnace. They recommend shovelling it down the gullet regardless of the body's condition.

Most athletes are still wrapped up in this old fallacy. Only the more informed realize the value of fasting both in training and racing. As Dr. Ernst van Aaken points out:

"The same powers are utilized in both training and healing," says author Ian Jackson. "In the first case, they transform health to superior health." (Stowe Photo)

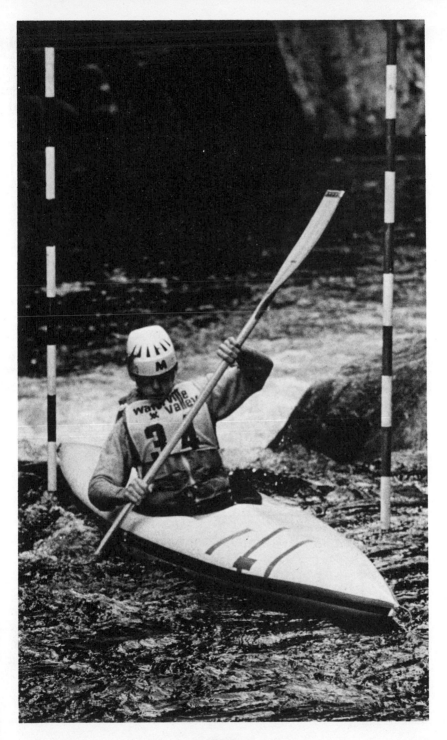

"The axiom that before a competition as little as possible should be taken remains valid. Certain experiments even point out that it is best to fast completely from the day before, because the body does not run on what it consumes just before the run, but with the reserves it has built up in months and years of long training, chiefly in the liver, musculature and hormones, as well as in the enzymes. Digestion shortly before or during a race wastes energy. In order to force the reserves of the liver and of the muscles to build up from the body substances and from surplus depots it is advisable, especially for the marathon runner, to put in occasional days of strict fasting, perhaps beginning the day before, covering the marathon distance at a slow pace on the following day."

Radical advice? It's all radical advice. Ignore it if you want. Ridicule it if you want. But remember, it might be true. And if that "might be" starts to bother you, read the hygienists, try their advice, and prove it for yourself.

GREEN POWER FOR ATHLETES

Like carrion crows, we live and feed on meat,
Regardless of the suffering and pain
We cause by doing so. If thus we treat
Defenseless animals for sport or gain,
How can we hope in this world to attain
The PEACE we say we are so anxious for?
We pray for it, o'er hecatombs of slain,
To God, while outraging the moral law,
Thus cruelty begets its offspring—War.

George Bernard Shaw

"It was too much for some of the visitors—the men would look at each other, laughing nervously, and the women would stand with hands clenched and the blood rushing to their faces, and the tears starting in their eyes."—Upton Sinclair, visit to a slaughterhouse, from *The Jungle*

Years ago vegetarianism was considered a nervous preoccupation of pipsqueaks—effete, shadowy intellectuals, mama's boys and

Malibu health freaks. There is some truth in this image: those who've felt most out-of-place in society have always sought solutions and company outside normal channels. Thus the health food movement and vegetarianism have been natural gathering places for the physically, mentally and emotionally "disabled."

"Natural foods" became hip when Madison Avenue took an interest in the commercial aspects of long hair and beads. Supermarkets now carry granola, herb shampoos and bread made with "all natural ingredients." Posh restaurants in urban centers do a big business in highly spiced and sauced vegetarian meals. Ralph Nader has embarrassed the FDA, and the ecology movement has prodded New York publishers to invest in books like *Diet for a Small Planet.*

There's not much real, ahem, meat for the athlete in all this frippery. But food reform's new social acceptance has made athletes more eager for information about the best fuels for athletic performance. *Bike World* editor George Beinhorn has been a cyclist, distance runner and vegetarian for seven years. He says, "I'm constantly surprised at the way cyclists and runners 'pick my brain' when they find out I'm a vegetarian. I belong to a large San Francisco distance running club, the Pamakids (Pa, Ma and Kids). We went out to a pizza parlor recently after the weekly club run and I had to answer spontaneous questions about vegetarianism for an hour. And it wasn't just idle curiosity—these people are really interested in improving their athletic 'high.' The same thing happened after I talked on diet at a Pedali Alpini cycling club meeting—the same intense interest."

For what it's worth, a great number of famous historical figures have been vegetarians: Plato, Diogenes, Pythagoras, the Buddha, Seneca, Virgil, Ovid, Horace, St. Paul, Jesus (cf. *The Essene Gospel of Peace*), Plutarch, Shakespeare, Da Vinci, Newton, Rousseau, Voltaire, Benjamin Franklin, Darwin, Emerson, Gen. William Booth, Thoreau, Shelley, Alexander Pope, Tagore, Tolstoy, H. G. Wells, Edison, Einstein, G. B. Shaw, Schweitzer, Gen. George Montgomery, Gandhi. It's estimated that the number of vegetarians in the US currently is between two and a half and three million (1969).

As Ralph Bircher pointed out, meat isn't essential. Further evidence of this comes to us from the physiology of the human body. Carnivores, omnivores (mixed meat and vegetable diet) and fruitarians in the animal kingdom are set apart by peculiarities in tooth structure and intestinal tract which correspond to the problems of eating and digesting the characteristic food of the animal's diet.

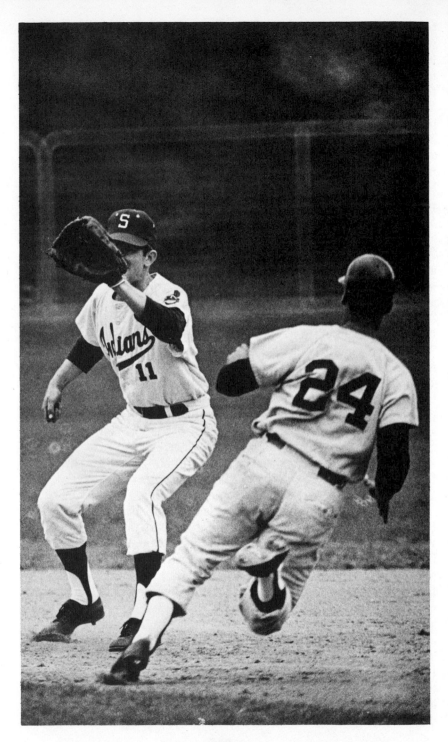

Meat decays quickly in the warmth of the intestinal tract. Thus carnivores have an intestinal tube only three times the length of their body, measured from mouth to anus. Meat-eaters' stomachs manufacture abundant hydrochloric acid, suitable for digesting bone and flesh. Herbivores (cattle, etc.) have several stomachs and an intestinal tract 10 times the length of their body. Their alkaline saliva contains ptyalin for the digestion of starches. Grains don't decay as rapidly as meat, so they don't form toxins of decomposition in the long intestinal tracts of these animals.

The digestive tract of the frugivorous (fruit-eating) animals is 12 times the length of their body. By this criterion, man is a frugivore.

Carnivores' teeth are made for stabbing, ripping and tearing their prey; omnivores have flat molars for grinding, as well as long canines; herbivores have grass-cutting and -grinding teeth, with broad, flat molars; and frugivores have pre-molars and molars suited to cracking nuts and grinding fruit and vegetables. Man's canine teeth "bear no real resemblance to the 'long and pointed stabbing weapons' found in both the natural carnivore and omnivore," according to Nathaniel Altman, whose book *Eating for Life* is an excellent source for prospective vegetarians.

Altman also points out that man's instincts are not those of a carnivore. A carnivore's mouth waters at the sight of fresh, raw meat and it pounces eagerly on the live animals who provide its food, eating their flesh raw. Man hides his slaughterhouses at the edges of his cities and has to disguise meat by cooking and spices before it passes the test of his sense of taste. Fruits, on the other hand, appeal to our senses of sight, smell and taste.

There are no pure fruit-eating animals in nature; all eat nuts, grains, leaves, roots and tubers as well. But our mainstay is fruit. "Nothing affords us more good eating pleasure than a rich, mellow apple, a luscious, well-ripened banana, a carefully-selected buttery, creamy, smooth avocado, or the wholesome, heart-warming goodness of a sweet grape. Real gustatory happiness is derived from the peach brought to the point of ripe perfection." Anyone who's finished a long, hard race or training session and has felt that intense, specific craving for fruit of all kinds and in great amounts knows Herbert Shelton isn't just weaving fantasies in his praise of fruit—*the* prime source of enzymes, vitamins and minerals for the athlete.

Vegetarian baseball players? Sounds heretical but people will do a lot for a result which they won't do merely to buck tradition, so we may see it.

Fruit is the easiest and most quickly-digested food of man, remaining only 30 minutes or so in the stomach, compared with as long as four hours for meat proteins; with its rich supply of natural sugars it is the ideal food for consumption before and during long events.

Altman gives five reasons why meat is not an optimal food:

1. **Putrefaction.** Animal flesh putrefies in a very short time. "Food experts generally agree that putrefaction has set in when a frankfurter's total bacteria count has reached 10 million per gram. With that as a yardstick, more than 40 percent of the samples we analyzed had begun to spoil. One sample tested out at 140 million bacteria per gram." (*Consumer Reports*, 2/72)

2. **Bodily poisons.** "Toxic wastes, including uric acid, are present in the blood and tissue, as also are dead and virulent bacteria, not only from the putrefactory process, but from animal diseases, such as hoof and mouth disease, contagious abortion, swine fever, malignant tumors, etc. ·Similarly, meat contains vaccines injected into the animals against prevalent diseases." (*Encyclopedia Britannica*)

3. **Pain poisoning.** "Just before and during the agony of being slaughtered, large quantities of adrenalin are forced through the entire body, thus pain-poisoning the entire carcass. Even the meat industry acknowledges that pre-slaughter psychological stress produces physical changes in the carcass . . . in a recent interview, a spokesman from the American Meat Institute conceded that there are many more implications to pain-poisoning which are yet to be understood." *(Eating for Life)*

4. **Chemical additives.** The list of chemicals being used in *all* meats currently sold in our markets is much too long to discuss in detail. Just one example is DES (diethylstilbestrol), which causes cattle and sheep to gain weight very quickly. Altman says: "The November 8, 1971 issue of *Newsweek* reports: 'There is mounting evidence for a link between DES and cancer . . . Some 75 percent of the 34 million beef cattle and 16 million sheep that wind up on American dinner tables each year have been fattened on feedlots where DES has been sprinkled on their fodder.'"

5. **Pesticides.** "Evidence presented at the International Symposium on Food Protection held at Iowa State University in 1962 showed that most of the DDT found in humans comes from meat and related products . . . the average concentration of DDT in the general population of the United States was 4.9 parts per million, while the average concentration found in those who abstain from meat was only 2.3 parts per million per person—less than half." *(Eating for Life)*

Consumer Reports said of federal meat inspection, which suffers notoriously from an inadequate staff of inspectors: "We found that one-eighth of the Federally inspected sausage and more than one-fifth of the other [non-Federally inspected] sausage contained insect fragments, larvae, rodent hairs and other kinds of filth . . . To put it bluntly, Federal inspection is evidently failing to do its job." (August 1968 issue, quoted in *Eating for Life*) The sausage tested by *CR* came from five widely separated states (New York, Pennsylvania, Illinois, New Mexico, California).

Considering these facts, it's not surprising that the vegetarian Seventh Day Adventists have 40% fewer heart and blood vessel diseases than the general population, and that cut-rate insurance is now being sold to vegetarians by a London firm.

Protein and vitamin B_{12}, as Dr. Hoyt pointed out, are the bugaboos of vegetarian diet. An excellent work on combining vegetable proteins for a full-value supply is *Diet for a Small Planet*. However, the need for eating combinations of protein foods is seriously questioned by hygienists who've had long, successful experience with diets in which only one protein is eaten at a time. The hygienists base their case on arguments like Herbert Shelton's: "Due to the fact that each separate kind of food determines a definite hourly rate of secretion and occasions characteristic limitations in the various powers of the [digestive] juices, foods requiring marked differences in the digestive secretions, as, for example, bread and flesh, certainly should not be consumed at the same meal." (*Food Combining Made Easy*)

While hygienists don't recommend combining two protein foods, they do recommend that "all kinds of non-starchy and succulent vegetables" be eaten with proteins, and in many cases these contain proteins that complement the amino acid deficiencies of the principle protein food of the meal.

As to the *amount* of food that must be eaten in order to provide minimum daily needs on a vegetarian diet, this has frequently been exaggerated. One health food store manager who frowns on vegetarianism told us, "You'd have to eat nuts all day to get enough protein." Her calculations were based on 75 grams and more per day which, as we've seen (Hoyt, Bircher), is far above true needs.

In fact, the MDR is filled by eating four slices of whole wheat bread and one pint of cow's or soya milk per day. One cup of almonds contains 30 grams of high-quality protein. It's been the experience of Herbert Shelton in over 50 years of nutrition research and practice that eating varied proteins *at different meals* instead of all at the same meal, and in the desirable combinations with vegetables, produces excellent health as tested over periods far longer than those in which a protein deficiency would show up.

The otherwise very useful book *Diet for a Small Planet* is also excessively calorie-conscious. Author Frances Lappé excluded pecans, almonds and other superb protein sources from her recommendations "because they contain too many calories for the amount of protein you get." This is very misleading. It is a curious and yet-unexplained fact that vegetarians can eat the same amount of calories as meat-eaters, and still gain much less weight. Hardinge and Stare found in their *Nutritional Studies of Vegetarians* that "'Pure' vegetarian men and women averaged 20 pounds less than the other two groups (meat-eaters and milk-and-egg-eating vegetarians), despite approximately the same caloric intakes and physical activities."

Bike World editor George Beinhorn experienced the same phenomenon: "When I gave up meat and started eating a diet of all-raw foods and raw milk, my weight dropped from 175 and stayed within a few pounds of 150. When I tried a pure vegan (no milk) diet using mainly nuts for protein, I immediately lost eight pounds more, though my caloric intake was about the same and I was exercising *less*."

Many economic forecasters see hard times ahead in this country, and a number of books have appeared concurrent with such predictions, on "saving money by using non-meat proteins." In an economic pinch, meat would certainly become the food of the rich, since the rancher produces beef on a low profit margin and an inflationary market would tempt him to get out of the business and raise seasonal crops. A depression would probably drive him to raise his own food and for the rest, just get what he could— eliminating the expensive worry of feeding cattle. Altman, in *Eating for Life,* quotes Dr. Aaron Altschul, a research chemist for the Department of Agriculture: "In terms of the average pounds of amino acids per acre, the soybean produces close to 17 lb. per acre compared with about two for milk and less than one for beef." (*Proteins: Their Chemistry and Politics*) Over half the harvested acreage in the US is planted to animal feed crops, and it's estimated that food production would quadruple if this land were used for direct food crops instead.

Muscle sports like water polo require no more protein than golf or croquet, according to researchers—and protein is protein, whether it comes from the plant that grew out of the ground, or the body of the animal that ate it. (John Marconi Photo)

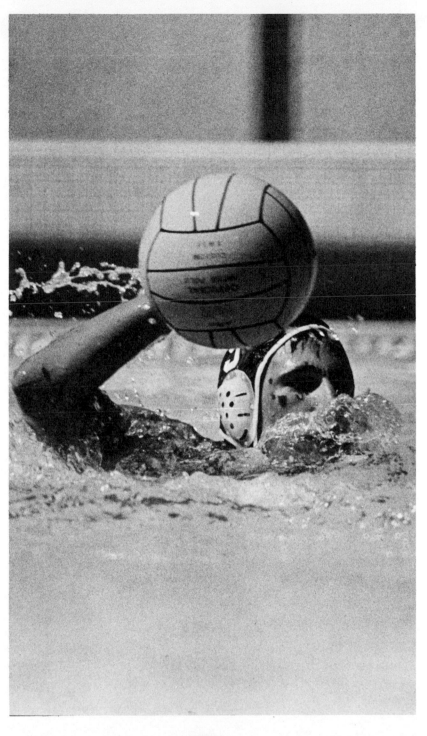

Meat is vastly more expensive than vegetable protein. A pound of soy flour in 1971 cost 11 cents, compared with 55 cents for hamburger, 65 cents for chicken, $1.20 for pork, and $1.50–$2.00 for steak and lamb chops. Sunflower and sesame seeds, the staple proteins in large areas of the world, are still around 80 cents a pound in the fancy retail packages (1974), while in bulk they're even cheaper. *Eating for Life* and *Diet for a Small Planet* give many suggestions for saving money on proteins.

A famous study done by Hindhede, Food Advisor to the Danish government during World War I, discovered that when meat and alcohol were in extremely short supply and the population got very little of these two products, the death rate per 1000 population fell to the lowest rate of any European country at any time. "I believe," said Hindhede, "I have shown that a diet containing a large amount of meat and eggs is dangerous to health." Frederick J. Stare, M.D., chairman of Harvard University's Department of Nutrition, has said, "There is nothing nutritionally wrong with vegetarian diets . . . Good vegetarian diets are very healthful." (*Ladies' Home Journal*, October 1971)

As Bircher points out, grains have been discovered to be a source of vitamin B_{12}, a deficiency of which was commonly feared in strict vegan diets containing no dairy products. Physiologist René Dubos points out in *Man Adapting* that many vegans live in good health on diets extremely low in any apparent sources of B_{12}: "A plausible explanation of this finding is that bacterial synthesis of the vitamin takes place in the intestine of these vegans, much as it does in sheep and other animals." Many find it difficult to adapt to a vegan diet, however, after years of eating meat and dairy products. Perhaps the solution lies in a gradual switch to lacto-vegetarian diet, then cautious experiments with veganism.

If this article has caught your interest in a meatless diet, we strongly recommend Nathaniel Altman's *Eating for Life* (Quest Books, Wheaton, Ill.) and the works of Herbert Shelton, especially *Orthotrophy, Vol. II* and *Food Combining Made Easy*.

Probably the biggest problem in giving up meat is social pressures against changing. We'll talk about these later.

We haven't mentioned moral arguments against killing animals, except in the quotes at the beginning of this article. We're limited here to matters more directly concerned with performance and health, but if you're interested in this question you'll find Altman's unemotional and concise discussion very informative.

TO EAT OR NOT TO EAT

Park Barner is an ultra-marathon runner with an adventurous spirit. During the week before the 1973 52½-mile London-to-Brighton run, Park decided to try what amounts to the opposite of carbohydrate loading. The 28-year-old Pennsylvanian drank only fruit juices during that week and took his last "food," except for water, 24 hours before the race. Park was astonished at the results: he experienced no glycogen "crash" during the race, and ran almost a half-hour faster than his previous best time for 50 miles. "Two weeks later, in the 36-miler," reports *Runner's World* magazine, "he used the same fasting technique. He passed the marathon (26 miles, 385 yards) within minutes of his best time at that distance, and went on another 10 miles at the same pace."

Ken Swenson similarly decided to "risk all" before the important 1972 Olympic trials meet. Like Park Barner, Ken only drank fruit juices during the seven days prior to his race. He ran a personal record at 800 meters and made the Olympic team.

Marathoner Ian Jackson fasted for seven days on light quantities of juices and water. During this week he ran 130 miles in training—almost 20 miles every day. Ian described his last run of 20 miles in *The Runner's Diet:* "Although the pace got hot, it was absurdly easy to stay with it. I remember experiencing a sense of calm detachment. My body was moving effortlessly, gliding along with no urging. Everything was smooth, mellow and peaceful. My senses were incredibly heightened, finely tuned in. I felt a natural unity with the dark trees and the drifting mist. The sighing of the wind in the pines, the clear bird calls and the occasional creaking of branches seemed to penetrate gently into the very center of my being. With a combination of elation and gratitude, I let my body move on while my mind and my senses touched their home."

In a *Runner's World* poll, it was found that 13% of the distance runners surveyed frequently fasted for one to three days on water and juices.

The Tarahumara indians of northern Mexico run kick-ball relays for 100 to 200 miles at a time. The races last up to two days. Physiologists estimate that these runs burn up over 10,000 calories, and yet the vegetarian Tarahumaras barely eat that much in a week. Their diet is quite high in carbohydrates and extremely low in protein. The indians eat no fat, eggs, potatoes or sweets for two to five days before their relays.

A recent *National Geographic* study found that people who live extremely long lives have several things in common, regardless of where they live. They eat lightly, exercise every day, and their diets contain little or no meat.

What is it about eating little and fasting? The ancient Olympians fasted regularly, and modern Olympic multiple gold medalist Murray Rose fasted before his '56 and '60 Olympic games wins.

It's immediately obvious that the body gets a rest while fasting. Herbert Shelton, in a brilliant book, *Fasting for the Renewal of Life*, says, "Estimates of the amount of work done and energy expended in the daily work of digesting and handling three meals are, of necessity, only approximations, but they reveal that digestion is real work. To cease eating for a time constitutes one of the surest means of rest."

Shelton has been conducting fasts and studying why fasting works for more than 50 years. What he's learned may help us understand why it works so well for the athlete, and how fasting can be best applied to improving athletic performance and health.

Word-of-mouth had it when we were children that a person couldn't live more than a week or so without food, and at most three days without water. Comedian Dick Gregory disproved this for all time with his widely publicized 40-day water fasts. But Gregory was no pioneer—some spiders have survived 17 months without food! Shelton talks at length about interesting historical fasts, many of which were undertaken as political protests. Sick animals hide and fast also, letting the body turn its energies to the process of elimination and healing.

Why don't we die when we go without food? A family who crashed their small plane in Alaska were snowbound without food for 40 days before they were able to walk out—in excellent condition.

Shelton explains what the body does when it's given no food:

"When either man or animal ceases to eat, no matter why, the demand for substance with which to maintain the structure and function of the vital tissues is thrown upon the reserves and expendables of the abstaining organism. It is only after these reserves and expendables are exhausted that the organized tissues are requisitioned as sources of nutritive material. When we fast, the functioning tissues must live upon something. Surpluses and stored materials (stored for just such emergencies) are called upon to supply nutriment for these functioning, therefore hungry, tissues. Some of these are oxidized to provide heat. The consequence is that the surpluses that are cluttering up the avenues of life are removed. The fasting organism nourishes its functioning tissues upon intrinsic nutrient stores and removes all accumulated and stored debris from its precincts."

Many old objections to fasting were based on post-mortem examinations of individuals who had *starved*. But Shelton points out that starvation does not begin with the first meal omitted, and that there are four stages which the organism undergoes when food is absent, only the *last* of which is actual starvation:

1. "The period of transition from a state of adequate feeding to the basal metabolism of fasting."

2. "A period that is characterized by a reduction of physiological activities to a minimum peculiar to the individual."

3. "This is merely a later phase of the second period and is not well marked-off."

4. "This final phase is marked by a predominance of pathological developments resulting from an exhaustion of reserves and of tissues."

These periods will begin at different times and have different durations, depending on the toxic conditions and stored reserves of the individual. Shelton has found in the thousands of long fasts he's conducted that hunger disappears after three to five days, and only after it returns again—which may be as long as a month—does *starvation* begin.

A gain in strength after ending the fast seems to be a common phenomenon. Many people undertaking fasts of several weeks or more mention feeling "strong as steel," even increasing in strength during the late stages of not eating, and after the fast is ended.

The how-to of fasting is basically quite simple, but it does involve considerations of your individual health. If you've had a terrible diet for years and suddenly go without food for 40 days, to give an extreme example with extreme consequences, you might run into a "toxic crisis": the eliminatory mechanisms may have more than they can handle at some point during their attempts to rid the body of poisons. If this happens it's good to have someone around who knows what's happening and what to do. Read Shelton's book before deciding on extreme measures.

How can you stand to be hungry for such a long time? A little-known secret of fasting is that hunger completely disappears in two to four days. People who fast regularly feel little or no

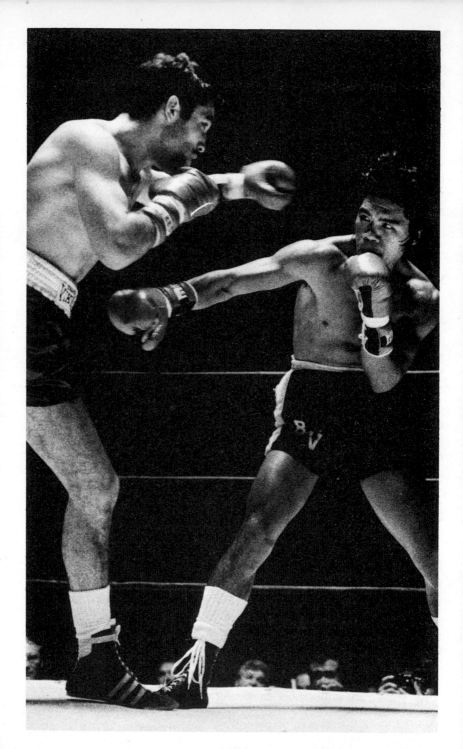

hunger at all from the moment they decide not to eat. Hunger in the first stages of a fast is 100% psychological. It is physiologically impossible to starve before reaching the skeleton stage, and real hunger—which as Shelton points out is a *mouth* sensation and not the "gnawing" in the stomach we often call hunger—rarely returns within the first two weeks. The body realizes at some point in the first four days that the eating cycle is broken, so it stops signalling for food.

What about vitamins? Shouldn't you take a supplement? Shelton says the body's supply of vitamins is adequate for a long fast. When the body decides it needs food once again, it signals you to feed it, by feelings of true hunger. In any case, as Shelton points out, when the amount of food taken in is decreased, the need for vitamins is correspondingly reduced.

In the first day or two of a fast you feel great energy—the result of giving the body a rest from shoving food through about 40 feet of tubing, plus all the chemical processes of digestion. "Fasting has been appropriately called a *rest of metabolism.* There is no doubt that the glands that are the chief agents of control of the metabolic processes are given a rest and thus permitted to normalize both their structures and their activities. There can be no doubt that this increased excretion is largely responsible for much of the benefit that flows from a period of abstinence."

The effects of fasting are limited by the inherent powers of your own individual organism. It won't make you a superman: "The fast may increase the efficiency of the organism, it cannot provide it with new powers."

"The changes that take place in one fasting are not confined to the mental outlook, the emotional life and the senses, but are seen in the whole of the body. Old accumulations are removed, toxins are expelled, secretions are normalized, the tissues are renewed, metabolism is rejuvenated, the individual fasts into newness of life. A properly conducted fast is indeed the *Great Preparation."* Not a bad way to go into a game or race.

"Fasting is merely a first step required by those who desire to recapture the joyous exuberance of life that our primeval ancestors knew. Their animation and zest has been lost in great degree, due to our loss of vigor and purity of life. To regain it requires that we cleanse our body of the debris that has accumulated as a consequence of a lifetime of unwholesome living."

Boxers like Ray Lunny (L) may fast to make a weight limit, but might also benefit from its cleansing effects.

Training or racing while on a fast runs contrary to the health benefits of the practice: "While fasting it is necessary to reduce stresses to a minimum, thus conserving the resources of the fasting organism—it is quite correct to say that stress factors are hurtful during a fast." Exercise checks elimination, lessening the fast's effects.

The athlete works untold hours training his heart, lungs, chemical metabolism, nerves and muscles to optimal efficiency. He or she is constantly improving on the execution of a magnificent design. It's like a brilliant automotive designer who's drawn up a racing motor far ahead of its time. That design is our individual potential. Engineers work for years, improving the materials available for the construction of a test engine. Even so do we constantly improve the quality of our bodies. But no engineer would ever dream of putting into this racing engine fuels that do not "burn clean," or sending it into a major competition with piston rings carbon-fouled, valves in need of grinding, and carburetor delivering an inefficient fuel/air mixture. Likewise, fasting is the body's way of cleaning itself out and setting its valves for optimal performance. "Fasting does not increase the possibilities of life, it only enables the body to realize them."

LOOKING FOR YOUR RAINBOW

Fight always for the highest attainable aim,
But never put up resistance in vain.

Hans Selye, M.D.

Herbert Shelton says it takes three to five years to change eating habits. Everybody has a unique eating pattern that works best for their own body, and it takes time to let the body adapt to new foods, time to find out what *your* body likes best, and time to replace old habits and tastes with new ones. Some people can never thrive on an all-raw foods diet; others can switch radically and never look back.

It takes time to learn to *like* new foods. Giving up everything you now eat and taking up a completely new diet with different tastes, textures, amounts and timing, is like grabbing a tiger by the tail. Those old habits have big muscles, and they're going to give you a battle, so it's better to teach the old animal one trick at a time. Here are some suggestions to make changing a little easier, based on our own experience.

Don't rush into this. Before you omit a single teaspoon of white sugar from your diet, you must know *why* you're doing it. You don't have to memorize scientific research papers. But you are inevitably going to fail unless you have two powerful allies: (1) diamond-hard, intelligent conviction that what you are doing is best; and (2) your own experience of what it feels like to eat well.

St. Francis called his body "Brother Donkey." What you have to do to get Brother Donkey to move is tempt him with carrots from the front while applying a good swift kick from behind. The carrots are tempting new ideas, and the experiences of other people. It's indispensable to keep a bushel or so of these on your bookshelf to nourish your motivation. The good swift kick is will power applied in short-term campaigns of good eating, to give yourself a taste for the benefits to be derived from change. When you experience the kind of energy and lightness that has you almost floating off the ground, you'll want more.

Take the long view. The best advice we've ever heard was: "No matter how many times you fall, pick yourself up, brush yourself off, and start over again." This isn't just useless homily, but is based on a deep truth. Ignorant people try once and then give up, rationalizing that they just weren't born with a strong will. But psychologists know that the will to accomplish something begins life like a little baby—a helpless, directionless wish. Feed it with inspiring ideas, give it the backbone of experience and reason, and it gradually grows into something different—dynamic volition. Volition is the mature stage of will power, which shows as repeated, undiscouraged actions toward an end.

No matter that you can't resist that marshmallow sundae. Think far ahead: "In five years, there's just *no way* I'm going to be prevented from enjoying fantastic health!" So wipe the syrup off your chin and keep feeding your mental "ball of string" with new facts about health and your own potential—until it's so huge there's no longer any room in your mind for wrong concepts and rationalization.

Feeling guilty is stupid, inefficient. Forget the past! It is not you. Start flexing your mental muscles and dry up spilled milk with the towel of new wisdom.

John Tilden, M.D., was one of Herbert Shelton's early teachers. Whenever Shelton made some dietary error or slip, Tilden would boom out exultantly: "I have learned to repent before I sin, and don't have to suffer remorse!" This is an expression of what's been called "Won't Power." If you stand there looking in the refrigerator while desperately trying to muster your reasons for not eating all that junk, next thing you know you'll be sitting at the table with a mouthful of food. Transactional psychology says that at different times people play roles of adult, parent and child toward themselves. When a child is strictly forbidden to do something harmful, it cries and screams. The loving parent remains adamant against harmful leniency. The child eventually faces the hard fact of abstinence and learns to live without. Later it realizes the great benefit and power it received through early discipline, and the great love of its parents in imposing restrictions. When you're tempted, immediately say, "No!" and *get away* from temptation. *Then* use your reason. The more you do this, the more powerful, free and happy you'll be.

Make simple changes at first. You can make tremendous first improvements in your diet with almost no noticeable changes in taste and amount. Most of your bad food has "healthy equivalents." Here are some ideas for gradual first steps:

● Cut out all white sugar and use only honey and dried fruits for sweetener and candy. As we saw earlier, so-called "brown," "raw" and "kleenraw" sugars are nothing but white sugar disguised in various ways. Your sense of taste will, in time, return to its natural state. White sugar will then taste noxious, sickly-sweet and repulsive. Fruit will taste like the nectar of the gods.

● Eat only 100% whole wheat products. Some breads are called "whole wheat" but contain white flour. Read the label. "Unbleached white flour" is almost as bad as ordinary white flour: it is just as effective in gumming up the intestines and preventing other foods from being properly absorbed. Many markets as well as health food stores stock 100% whole wheat spaghetti, granola, crackers and cookies, as well as other unrefined, sugarless grain products.

● Cook vegetables lightly, and never eat them without also eating a raw salad at the same meal. Try spinach or Swiss chard cooked this more healthy way: boil about an inch of water in a covered pot. Put in a big gob of greens and peek under the lid every five seconds or so. The instant they "collapse," take them out and eat them with a light sprinkling of lemon juice and a little butter or oil. You'll never eat that putrid mess known as "cream spinach" again. Better yet, get a special pot for steaming where the vegetable remains above the boiling water.

● Eat little beef and pork, substituting fish and chicken and vegetable proteins. Some vegetarian recipe books have recipes for taste-alike all-vegetable meat substitutes. Artificial meats are sold in the health food sections of many markets nowadays.

- Learn to never overeat. Some of the long-lived people in the *National Geographic* study had atrocious diets, but all ate very little. Experiment with eating less, making mental notes of how you feel. More than anything else, cut down on fats, proteins and carbohydrates. These are the most difficult-to-digest foods, the most apt to make you feel sluggish.

- Organize your eating so you get all the essentials every day. A body without all the proper nutrients is like a cement wall without lime: it looks o.k. for awhile, but it eventually crumbles.

- Explore. Eating more "alive" foods should be an adventurous, fun thing. Returning to the natural tastes of primitive man is an immensely renewing experience. Several vegetarians we know say their tastes have become so "naturalized" that a bowl of romaine lettuce, raw spinach leaves, sprouts and tomatoes with a little orange juice sprinkled on it is one of the most mouthwatering delights they can imagine.

- Study food combining. This alone works wonders, especially if you have unexplained digestive problems. Shelton's *Food Combining Made Easy* is a fine book on the topic, and on nutrition in general.

If you get hooked on the idea of changing, you may want to do extensive reading. Watch out for bad books. Some authors do a remarkable job of describing the benefits of food reform, while advocating diets that in the long run are less than optimal. "Miracle food" books sing the glories of seaweed, honey, vitamin E, yeast, ginseng and other single items. They're all suspect: it's a universal principle of nutrition that any one food is only effective to the extent that it's supplied in an otherwise full-value diet. Excess vitamins, as Creig Hoyt told us, are either eliminated in the urine, are toxic, or throw the overall vitamin balance out of whack.

One of the interesting things about the books of Herbert Shelton is that he views fasting and raw food diet—which he strongly advocates—in perspective as only one part of the healthy life. Exercise, emotional stability, rewarding work, etc. are essential too, according to the hygienic system.

One-sided books do have their uses; they can motivate you by their vivid descriptions and tales of personal experiences and cures, but beware of one-sidedness, which can appear under a cloak of seeming innocence. One example of a dangerous but nice-sounding practice is the great quantity of fresh fruit and vegetable juices recommended by some books. When you consider that it takes about 10 carrots to make one large glass of carrot juice, it's easy to see that this can lead to "metabolic gluttony" and hypervitaminosis, upsetting the balance of chemical elements in the body. There are no health food miracles. No food or drug ever does or ever has performed a "cure." The human body heals itself, given usable amounts of clean fuels.

If you decide to give up coffee, salt, meat or any other harmful stimulant, you'll feel low for a few days. This doesn't mean the whole diet reform thing is hogwash—the body is just rectifying a chemically stimulated condition, immediately dumping some of the accumulated poisons. Bieler's *Food is Your Best Medicine* will give you a lot of supportive information to help you understand what's going on.

An eating diary is as useful as a training diary if you're really serious about changing. It prevents "convenient" lapses of memory, shows cumulative trends, helps you spot food items that are giving you digestive trouble, stimulates your pride in setting personal records, helps control eating between meals, and makes it hard for your conscience to relax or "take time out." We've found 3 x 5 cards convenient, kept in a small file box. You write the date in the upper right hand corner and just write down times and food eaten during the day, carrying the card around in a shirt pocket or purse. Start now. So what if you haven't got anything pure and wonderful to record? All the more reason for keeping a record . . . you'll become aware of the volume of junk in your diet and feel motivated to change.

Become consumer-aware. Take a look at the immense amount of advertising you're paying for when you buy boxed, processed and prettified trash. One of the reasons fresh raw foods aren't popular is that they receive almost no advertising. There's no way the big so-called "food manufacturers" can enrich, improve, pasteurize or substitute for nature's product. The Nader Group's *Chemical Feast* reminds us continually that those boxes and bottles that look so neat and pretty on the supermarket shelves have not been designed as a service to the shopper at all, but in effect to fleece him: "When one considers the crudeness of the food industry's power-flexing in the field of food standards, consumer boycotts and pickets seem quite reasonable." More effective, certainly, is gradually learning to "shop aware." The shopping

Everybody loves a shotputter, but the spectator's definition of health is beginning to differ from the athlete's. (Mark Shearman)

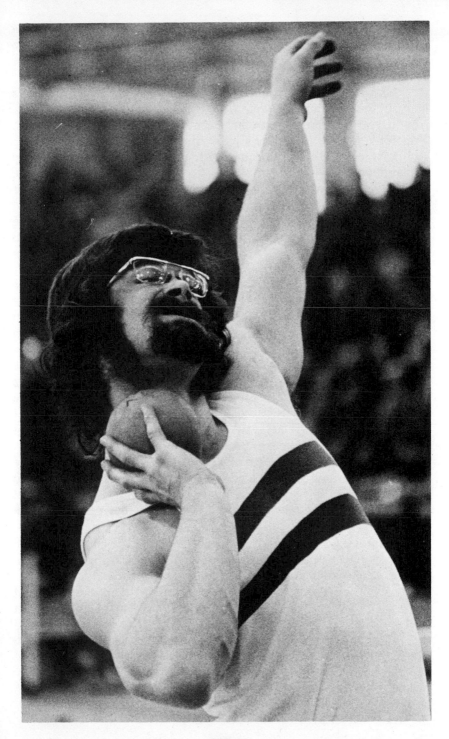

dollar speaks much more forcefully than government coercion—consider the new "natural food" lines being marketed by some big companies. Be your own advocate: if you don't take care of you, who will?

One final note on social pressures. Your family and friends may show annoying but well-intended concern: "You'll get sick. How'll you get enough protein? America wasn't built on carrots. You look terrible." There's only one solution to the problem: stubbornness. Make them live with you as you are. They may applaud your "wise decision" to slip back into irrational habits, but they won't hold your hand or experience your painful loss of health when overtaxed organs start to go.

You often can't avoid family and associates, but there's one type who's no friend at all and should definitely be shunned. Bob Dylan defined him well: "While one who sings with his tongue on fire/Gargles in the rat-race choir/Bent out of shape from society's pliers/Cares not to come up any higher/But rather get you down in the hole that he's in . . ." Philosopher Alan Watts remarked that one-upmanship is the single most universal negative human trait. Few are so inwardly honest with themselves that they can resist stealing a little cheap glory at their "friends'" expense—chopping off others' heads so they can feel taller. If you have friends who sincerely rejoice in your successes and never condone your errors and slips, consider them powerful allies in the battle to improve. Company is stronger than will power.

Athletes tend to be a little bit elitist. We know we've got something most people don't understand, and we think it's better. Athletes can talk on a level of experience for which the average person has no concepts. One way or another, we've all come to athletics and have become addicted to it because it helps us feel our own existence more keenly: something the passive person never knows.

Improving the quality of what you eat leads to more than just higher scores and faster racing. Athletics brings *new* complexes of experience . . . this is the unspoken secret we share. Similarly, pure foods, fasting and regulating the amount you eat renew all your senses and deepen the qualities of all your perceptions.

Buoyant, playful energy is supposed to be lost with childhood. It can be recovered—through exercise, as we've all found out—and by repairing the damage of putting improper fuels into this joyous machine.

Suggested Reading

If you'd like more information about nutrition and diet, we recommend the following books. You can try looking for these at your local bookstore, but will probably have better luck ordering directly from us. Just use the address given below, and add 15 cents per title postage and handling.

THE RUNNER'S DIET. The long-awaited guide to the feeding and watering of runners. Suggests ways to improve performance through dietary control, weight watching, proper drinking habits. Based on the latest scientific data and tested by runners themselves. 1972 paperback, 84 pp., ill., $1.95.

FOOD COMBINING MADE EASY, Herbert Shelton. Learn the correct food combining methods which can lead to improved endurance and strength based on total body usage of everything you eat. 1951 paperback, 76 pp., $1.95.

SUPERIOR NUTRITION, Herbert Shelton. A guide to rational and correct vegetarianism which can lead you to the enjoyment of the full benefits of a vegetarian diet, as proved by several of the world's leading endurance athletes. Discover a diet that's easy on your pocketbook and generous to your performances. 1951 paperback, 200 pp., $3.95.

BODY POLLUTION, Gary Null. A penetrating look at the foods and other substances we take into our bodies—how the poisons they contain can pollute our vital systems and destroy our health—and an alternative program of natural nutrition. 1973 hardback, 228 pp., $5.95.

FASTING FOR THE RENEWAL OF LIFE, Herbert Shelton. New book detailing what happens when the body is fasting. Shows the benefits of renewal and healing that fasting brings. 1973 paperback, $2.25.

HEALTH IS YOUR BIRTHRIGHT, Are Waerland. The methods of the world-famous Waerland system of healthful living are revealed in this book. An excellent source of food-as-therapy information. 1969 paperback, 88 pp., ill., $2.25.

World Publications, P.O. Box 366, Mountain View, CA 94040

THE VALUES OF FOODS

DAIRY PRODUCTS	MEASURE	WEIGHT grams	FOOD ENERGY Calories	PROTEIN grams	FAT grams	CALCIUM milli-grams	IRON milli-grams	VITAMIN A Int'l Units	VITAMIN B1 milli-grams	VITAMIN B2 milli-grams	VITAMIN B3 milli-grams	VITAMIN C milli-grams
MILK												
Cow's milk (whole fluid)	1 c.	244	160	9	9	288	0.1	350	0.07	0.41	0.2	2
Cow's milk (nonfat dry)	1 c.	104	375	37	1	1,345	.6	30	.36	1.85	.9	7
Soybean powd. (low fat dry)	1 c.	100	250	52	5.6	244	13.0	70	1.10	.35	2.9	—
CHEESE												
Cheddar cheese	1 oz.	28	115	7	9	213	.3	370	.01	.13	trace	0
Cottage cheese (creamed)	1 c.	245	260	33	10	230	.7	420	.07	.61	.2	0
Processed cheese (American)	1 oz.	28	105	7	9	198	.3	350	.01	.12	trace	0
CREAM												
Half and half	1 c.	242	325	8	28	261	.1	1,160	.07	.39	.1	2
Ice cream (10% fat)	1 c.	133	255	6	14	194	.1	590	.05	.28	.1	1
EGGS												
Eggs, large whole	each	50	80	6	6	27	1.1	590	.05	.15	trace	0

MEAT, POULTRY, FISH

	Measure	Grams	Calories	Protein	Fat	Calcium	Iron	Vit. A	Thiamine	Riboflavin	Niacin	Vit. C
MEAT												
Beef, ground & broiled	3 oz.	85	245	21	17	9	2.7	30	.07	.18	4.6	—
Beef steak, broiled sirloin	3 oz.	85	330	20	27	9	2.5	50	.05	.16	4.0	—
Frankfurter, heated	each	56	170	7	15	3	.8	—	.08	.11	1.4	—
Pork chops, cooked	3.5 oz.	98	260	16	21	8	2.2	0	.63	.18	3.8	—
Veal cutlet, cooked	3 oz.	85	185	23	9	9	2.7	—	.06	.21	4.6	—
POULTRY												
Chicken, flesh only, broiled	3 oz.	85	115	20	3	8	1.4	80	.05	.16	7.4	—
FISH												
Haddock, breaded, fried	3 oz.	85	140	17	5	34	1.0	—	.03	.06	2.7	2
Tuna, canned in oil,	3 oz.	85	170	24	7	7	1.6	70	.04	.10	10.1	—
DRY BEANS, PEAS, NUTS												
Almonds, shelled, whole	1 c.	142	850	26	77	332	6.7	0	.34	1.31	5.0	trace
Beans, great north., cooked	1 c.	180	210	14	1	90	4.9	0	.25	.13	1.3	0
Beans, lima, cooked	1 c.	190	260	16	1	55	5.9	0	.25	.11	1.3	0
Beans, navy, cooked	1 c.	190	225	15	1	95	5.1	0	.27	.13	1.3	0
Cashews, roasted	1 c.	140	785	24	64	53	5.3	140	.60	.35	2.5	—
Coconut, fresh shredded	1 c.	130	450	5	46	17	2.2	0	.07	.03	.7	4
Cowpeas, cooked, drained	1 c.	248	190	13	1	42	3.2	20	.41	.11	1.1	trace
Lentils, dry, cooked	1 c.	250	265	20	trace	68	5.3	150	.93	.55	5.0	—
Peanuts, roasted, halves	1 c.	144	840	37	72	107	3.0	—	.46	.19	24.7	0
Peanut butter	1 Tb.	16	95	4	8	9	.3	—	.02	.02	2.4	0
Peas, split, dried, cooked	1 c.	250	290	20	1	28	4.2	100	.37	.22	2.2	—
Pecans, halves	1 c.	108	740	10	77	79	2.6	140	.93	.14	1.0	2
Soybeans, dried, cooked	1 c.	180	208	18	9	117	4.3	48	.34	.14	1.0	0
Walnuts, black, chopped	1 c.	126	790	26	75	trace	7.6	380	.28	.14	.9	—

	MEASURE	WEIGHT	FOOD ENERGY	PROTEIN	FAT	CALCIUM	IRON	VITAMIN A	VITAMIN B1	VITAMIN B2	VITAMIN B3	VITAMIN C
		grams	calories	grams	grams	milli-grams	milli-grams	Int'l Units	milli-grams	milli-grams	milli-grams	milli-grams
Asparagus pieces, cooked	1 c.	145	30	3	trace	30	.9	1,310	.23	.26	2.0	38
Beans, green, cooked	1 c.	125	30	2	trace	63	.8	680	.09	.11	.6	15
Bean sprouts, mung, cooked	1 c.	125	35	4	trace	21	1.1	30	.11	.13	.9	8
Beets, cooked, sliced	1 c.	170	55	2	trace	24	.9	30	.05	.07	.5	10
Beet greens, cooked	1 c.	145	25	3	trace	114	2.8	7,400	.10	.22	.4	22
Broccoli, cooked	1 c.	155	40	5	1	136	1.2	3,880	.14	.31	1.2	140
Brussels sprouts, cooked	1 c.	155	55	7	1	50	1.7	810	.12	.22	1.2	135
Cabbage, raw, coarse shred	1 c.	70	15	1	trace	34	.3	90	.04	.04	.2	33
Carrots, raw	each	50	20	1	trace	18	.4	5,500	.03	.03	.3	4
Cauliflower, cooked, buds	1 c.	120	25	3	trace	25	.8	70	.11	.10	.7	66
Celery, large stalk	each	40	5	trace	trace	16	.1	100	.01	.01	.1	4
Corn, sweet, cooked	1 ear	140	70	3	1	2	.5	310	.09	.08	1.0	7
Cucumbers, raw, pared	each	207	30	1	trace	35	.6	trace	.07	.09	.4	23
Dandelion greens, cooked	1 c.	180	60	4	1	252	3.2	21,060	.24	.29	–	32
Kale, stems, leaves, cooked	1 c.	110	30	4	1	147	1.3	8,140	–	–	–	68
Lettuce, iceberg,	1 head	454	60	4	trace	91	2.3	1,500	.29	.27	1.3	29
Mustard greens, cooked	1 c.	140	35	3	1	193	2.5	8,120	.11	.19	.9	68
Onions, raw	each	110	40	2	trace	30	.6	40	.04	.04	.2	11
Parsley, raw, chopped	1 Tb.	4	trace	trace	trace	8	.2	340	trace	.01	trace	7
Parsnips, cooked	1 c.	155	100	2	1	70	.9	50	.11	.12	.2	16
Peas, green, cooked	1 c.	160	115	9	1	37	2.9	860	.44	.17	3.7	33

Food	Measure											
Peppers, sweet, raw	each	74	15	1	trace	7	.5	310	.06	.06	.4	94
Potatoes, baked, medium	each	99	90	3	trace	9	.7	trace	.10	.04	1.7	20
Radishes, small raw	each	10	1	trace	trace	3	.1	trace	trace	trace	trace	2
Spinach, cooked	1 c.	180	40	5	1	167	4.0	14,580	.13	.25	1.0	50
Squash, winter, baked	1 c.	205	130	4	1	57	1.6	8,610	.10	.27	1.4	27
Sweet potatoes, baked	each	110	155	2	1	44	1.0	8,910	.10	.07	.7	24
Tomatoes, raw	each	200	40	2	trace	24	.9	1,640	.11	.07	1.3	42
Tomato juice, canned	1 c.	243	45	2	trace	17	2.2	1,940	.12	.07	1.9	39
Turnips, cooked, diced	1 c.	155	35	1	trace	54	.6	trace	.06	.08	.5	34
Turnip greens, cooked	1 c.	145	30	3	trace	252	1.5	8,270	.15	.33	.7	68

FRUITS AND FRUIT PRODUCTS

Food	Measure											
Apples, raw	each	150	70	trace	trace	8	.4	50	.04	.02	.1	3
Apple juice, bottled/canned	1 c.	248	120	trace	trace	15	1.5	–	.02	.05	.2	2
Applesauce, canned, unsw.	1 c.	244	100	1	trace	10	1.2	100	.05	.02	.1	2
Apricots, dried, uncooked	1 c.	150	390	8	1	100	8.2	16,350	.02	.23	4.9	19
Apricot nectar, canned	1 c.	251	140	1	trace	23	.5	2,380	.03	.03	.5	8
Avocados, California, raw	each	284	370	5	37	22	1.3	630	.24	.43	3.5	30
Bananas, raw	each	175	100	1	trace	10	.8	230	.06	.07	.8	12
Blackberries, raw	1 c.	144	85	2	1	46	1.3	290	.05	.06	.5	30
Blueberries, raw	1 c.	140	85	1	1	21	1.4	140	.04	.08	.6	20
Cantaloupe, raw	each	770	120	2	trace	54	1.6	13,080	.16	.12	2.4	126
Dates, pitted, cut	1 c.	178	490	4	1	105	5.3	90	.16	.17	3.9	0
Figs, dried, large	each	21	60	1	trace	26	.6	20	.02	.02	.1	0
Grapefruit, raw, pink	each	482	100	2	trace	40	1.0	1,080	.10	.04	.4	88
Grapefruit juice, canned	1 c.	247	100	1	trace	20	1.0	20	.07	.04	.4	84
Grapes, raw, American type	1 c.	153	65	1	1	15	.4	100	.05	.03	.2	3
Lemons, raw	each	110	20	1	trace	19	.1	10	.03	.01	.1	39
Olives, green, pickled	each	4	4	trace	trace	2	.1	10	–	–	–	–

	MEASURE	WEIGHT grams	FOOD ENERGY calories	PROTEIN grams	FAT grams	CALCIUM milli-grams	IRON milli-grams	VITAMIN A Int'l Units	VITAMIN B1 milli-grams	VITAMIN B2 milli-grams	VITAMIN B3 milli-grams	VITAMIN C milli-grams
Oranges, raw	each	180	65	1	trace	54	.5	260	.13	.05	.5	66
Orange juice, fresh	1 c.	248	110	2	1	27	.5	500	.22	.07	1.0	124
Papayas, raw, cubed	1 c.	182	70	1	trace	36	.5	3,190	.07	.08	.5	102
Peaches, raw, medium	each	114	35	1	trace	9	.5	1,320	.02	.05	1.0	7
Pears, raw	each	182	100	1	1	13	.5	30	.04	.07	.2	7
Pineapple, raw, diced	1 c.	140	75	1	trace	24	.7	100	.12	.04	.3	24
Plums, raw	each	60	25	trace	trace	7	.3	140	.02	.02	.3	3
Raisins, seedless	1 c.	165	480	4	trace	102	5.8	30	.18	.13	.8	2
Raspberries, red, raw	1 c.	123	70	1	1	27	1.1	160	.04	.11	1.1	31
Strawberries, raw, capped	1 c.	149	55	1	1	31	1.5	90	.04	.10	1.0	88
Tangerines, raw, medium	each	116	40	1	trace	34	.3	360	.05	.02	.1	27
Watermelon, 4" x 8" wedge	each	925	115	2	1	30	2.1	2,510	.13	.13	.7	30
SUGARS, SWEETS												
Honey, strained or extracted	1 Tb.	21	65	trace	0	1	.1	0	trace	.01	.1	trace
Sugar, brown	1 c.	220	280	0	0	187	7.5	0	.02	.07	.4	0
Sugar, white, granulated	1 c.	200	770	0	0	0	.2	0	0	0	0	0
GRAIN PRODUCTS												
Barley, pearled, light, unc.	1 c.	200	700	16	2	32	4.0	0	.24	.10	6.2	0
Bread, white, enriched	1 lb.	454	1,225	39	15	381	11.3	trace	1.13	.95	10.9	trace

Food	Measure										
Bread, whole wheat	1 lb.	454	1,100	48	14	449	13.6	trace	1.18	.54	12.7	trace
Cornmeal, whole ground	1 c.	122	435	11	5	24	2.9	620	.46	.13	2.4	0
Graham crackers	each	7	28	1	1	3	.1	0	trace	.01	.1	0
Macaroni, enriched, cooked	1 c.	130	190	6	1	14	1.4	0	.23	.14	1.8	0
Oatmeal/rolled oats, cooked	1 c.	240	130	5	2	22	1.4	0	.19	.05	.2	0
Rice, brown, cooked	1 c.	205	238	5	1	24	1.0	0	.18	.04	2.8	0
Rice, enriched white, cooked	1 c.	205	225	4	trace	21	1.8	0	.23	.02	2.1	0
Whole wheat flour	1 c.	120	400	16	2	49	4.0	0	.66	.14	5.2	0
White flour, enriched	1 c.	115	420	12	1	18	3.3	0	.51	.30	4.0	0
Soybean flour, low fat	1 c.	120	425	52	8	315	10.9	96	1.00	.42	3.1	0
Wheat germ, raw	1 c.	100	363	27	11	72	9.4	0	2.01	.68	4.2	0

FATS AND OILS

Food	Measure										
Butter, regular, stick	½ c.	113	810	1	92	23	0	3,750	–	–	–	0
Cooking fats: lard	1 c.	205	1,850	0	205	0	0	0	0	0	0	0
Vegetable fats	1 c.	200	1,770	0	200	0	0	0	0	0	0	0
Margarine, regular, stick	½ c.	113	815	1	92	23	0	3,750	–	–	–	0
Oils, safflower	1 c.	220	1,945	0	220	0	0	0	0	0	0	0
Yeast, brewer's dry	1 Tb.	8	25	3	trace	17	1.4	trace	1.25	.34	3.0	trace

Index